A pocket guide to your pregnancy

How to become your own birth Doula

Lucy Bear

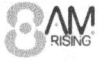

A pocket guide to your pregnancy:
How to become your own Birth Doula

Notice

The information provided in this book is not intended as a substitute for any treatment prescribed by your doctor. The information is not intended as medical advice nor is it meant to treat or diagnose any disease or mental disorder. If you have any medical problems, please seek competent medical help. This is not a medical manual; always seek the advice of your doctor.

Copyright © 2023 by Lucy Bear

All rights reserved. No part of this book may be reproduced in any manner whatsoever without written permission except in the case of brief quotations embodied in critical articles and reviews.

First Printing, 2022

To my son Marc Angelo

The book took shape from the moment you joined me to co-create the contents. You demystified the process of traveling deep inside to uncover the creative being that lives in all of us. The content is infused with your tender inspiration and magical eloquence. You will continue to nurture and inspire those who are yet to come. I am truly blessed and honored to be your mother. Everyone who knows you will agree! Thank you for your insight, patience and endurance.

To my Three Bears....

"...who else but you
please tell me who else
can ever take your place

now give yourself a smile
what is the worth of a diamond
If it doesn't shine

how can I ever put a price
on the diamond that you are
you are the entire treasure of the house"

—The Spiritual Poems of Rumi: Translated by Nader Khalili

CONTENTS

1. An Introduction to Our Expert—You ... 1
2. Let's Get Started ... 4
3. Riley's Story ... 12
4. An Amazing Transformation ... 17
5. A Journey Back to Your Own Beginning ... 21
6. What Are My Values? ... 34
7. Inspiring New Thoughts ... 38
8. Journaling ... 47
9. Affirmations ... 50
10. Relaxation ... 54
11. Preparations to Be a Great Dad ... 56
12. Making Changes as a Couple ... 61
13. Working on Your Relationship ... 68

CONTENTS

14 | Visualize Your Dreams and Goals 77
15 | Hypnobirthing 79
16 | The Benefits of Organizing Your Family and Friends 82
17 | Assert Yourself 88
18 | A Recap 89
19 | Your Body Is Changing—Are You Going to Change? 94
20 | The Benefits of Exercise 103
21 | What to Consider before Preparing Your Birth Plan 106
22 | Create Your Birth Plan 120
23 | Postpartum Essential List 124
24 | The Three Stages of Labor 128
25 | Postpartum 132
26 | Breastfeeding 135
27 | Bathing Baby 138
28 | Diapers 142

CONTENTS

29 | Postpartum Depression — Moms and Dads 146

30 | Self-Love and Self-Awareness 150

ABOUT THE AUTHOR 154

1

An Introduction to Our Expert—You

I am here to remind you that when it comes to yourself, you are the expert. There is no one who knows you better! There is no one better equipped to answer your questions than you. I can recall times when I've found myself anxiously lying in bed, thinking. Pondering and gestating the many steps which I thought I had to take in order to feel better about myself. From an early age, there are cumulative pressures asking us to be responsible, to finish school, to keep a job, and to follow the "normal" social path that will help sustain ourselves in the world. But, unsurprisingly, following this path alone does not prepare us for the challenges of a constantly changing world.

During our formative years, we spend much of our lives aspiring towards predictable and stable goals. Globally, we are currently witnessing downsizing, outsourcing, and a collapse of almost everything that we have invested and believed in. These changes have been further amplified by the removal of various constructs that enable and support our modern lifestyles. These events serve to accelerate us in a direction of awakening a deeper curiosity. My hope is that this spark will foster a desire for wholeness, and move us back towards our true selves.

A reflection of our true self allows us to be playful and creative, while also being resilient and well-adjusted. We have become comfortable with predictability and conformity, following a life recipe that brings repetitive results, but not necessarily our desired outcome. Changes to our normal daily life and work have forcibly imposed a self-introspection. Suddenly, we are confronted with the idea of having to solely take care of ourselves. Now is a good time to change anything that has not been working for you. Life is designed to connect us to our heart-led purpose. Challenges are always present. They are not intended to diminish us. Rather we can use these experiences to inspire personal growth and new ideas.

The Birth of a New Idea

Dana Raphael, a renowned and outspoken anthropologist, studied and explored our perceptions around breastfeeding. Her own devastation over not being able to breastfeed her son inspired her campaign and movement. Dana found that breastfeeding was more successful in some cultures. She also discovered that our methods for caring for expecting mothers, both before and after childbirth, were different across much of the world. For example, in parts of Asia and Latin America, there is a forty-day resting period for new mothers. In this protective environment, a mother is cared for and encouraged to eat special meals to help her regain her strength. Families share their knowledge about how to care for the baby. The mother refrains from household chores in order for her to solely concentrate on her well-being, and to feed the baby. The purpose of this supportive care is to "mother the mother," as Raphael put it.

Distance, lack of family support, work, divorce, and family disagreements can change the way we approach life. These circumstances often have a way of influencing our decisions. We can, however, make a choice and take steps to create healthier behaviors for ourselves. In this way, we are able to achieve a better outcome during birth, and strive to create a better environment for our children. Dr. Raphael told of a conversation with an elderly Greek woman, centering on intergenerational guidance and care of mothers. "You are describing a Doula," the woman explained to Dr. Raphael. The role of a Doula is as a non-medical caregiver who supports mothers during pregnancy, birth, and after childbirth. The Doula can be there to assist the mother, make her feel safe or comfortable, and complement any medical care given by a health professional. Whether you have access to a support person in your life, or not, I hope this book can guide you to become your own Doula.

2

Let's Get Started

Congratulations! If you have just picked up this book, I suspect that the good news has already reached you. You are exploding with excitement and planning the perfect pregnancy while also dealing with nausea, taste aversions, intense smells, and fatigue. While you are adjusting to your altered senses, your partner is also trying to process the changes to your mood, cravings, and requests. For example, your partner could find it daunting to locate a restaurant with a good menu and an even better bathroom to suit your frequent visits! If you are feeling lightheaded or teary, there is no point in trying to resist your body's prompting. Pregnancy is an emotional time. Your story is going to keep unfolding and you will continue to surprise yourself.

Your new role as a parent has been created and your ideas may change. Holding on to the past is like clinging to a false perspective. Start seeing situations in light of the future.

If there are two opinions or conflicting decisions, I hope that you will have the satisfaction of dissolving them in equal measure. Adapting will require mutual understanding, respecting, nurturing, listening, co-operating, sharing, as well as figuring out ways to negotiate and resolve problems.

It is astonishing how two people with different ideas around the same matter can become incomprehensible strangers. Alfred Korzybski was a Polish-born American independent scholar who is credited with developing the field of general semantics. His Law of Individuality states that "no two persons, or situations, or stages of processes are the same in all details." General semantics is a discipline and/or methodology intended to improve the ways people interact with their environment and with one another, especially through training in the critical use of words and other symbols. His Law of Individuality is paramount to navigating all the changes ahead.

I can still remember my own excitement and shock during my first pregnancy. While all these feelings are a normal initial response, I hope that they transition for you to an open-minded and inspired approach to parenthood.

Pregnancy Is Like a Marathon

How long does it take to prepare for and finish a marathon? This may seem like a strange question to ask in a book about pregnancy and childbirth, but preparing for a marathon requires the same significant amount of time to build a level of confidence to perform well. How someone performs in a marathon will depend on multiple factors: course difficulty, distance, hydration, nutrition, exercise, and how well the body adapts. Having the right equipment, preparing both mentally and physically, rewarding oneself with rest, relaxation, and perhaps a massage, will help contribute to success.

Instead of being in turmoil throughout the process, athletes make logistical preparations for any event. Most will confess that it was difficult in the beginning, and in order to achieve success, they had to also develop their mental focus. The more you practice something, the more automatic the response becomes. Athletes work with determination to achieve a desired result.

Most team players are fully engaged in the work, have a "can do" attitude, take the initiative to offer help, and they can count on reliability and commitment from the whole team. They feel safe enough to perform in a team without glancing over their shoulder, feeling vulnerable, or expecting trouble.

Even after intense preparation, life can be full of changes and surprises. There are obstacles and certain conditions beyond our control that could affect the course. Intense heat, heavy rain, and strong wind could hamper and disrupt a planned victory. If an athlete's thoughts are distracted and focused on the unpleasant conditions, it could deter their performance, make them feel anxious, and they may cave in.

I am here to encourage you and offer exercises that can help break through some of your self-imposed limitations. This guide can be used to prepare for the mental, emotional, and physical challenges ahead. That way, you will persevere and approach any situation with much more energy, confidence, and motivation. Along the pregnancy path, you can examine any mistakes or decisions in order to improve your experience. This event should not be seen as a setback or an interference. Instead, use it as a way to find solutions and bring clarity. It takes courage to fantasize about succeeding. Yet this is a clear indication of how your thoughts literally shape the world around you.

Pregnancy & Stress

Your brain is always busy. Evaluating, judging, and regulating your heartbeat, along with a thousand other micro-processes. We are unaware as most of these routine functions are being continually self-managed.

These processes occur automatically, such as breathing. At the same time, your beliefs structure your life. What if I told you that your body is already acting and performing according to your thoughts and emotions? If you are tense, fearful, angry, frustrated at work, under pressure to meet deadlines, and financially stressed, your brain becomes hardwired with an alarm system for your protection. Under these conditions, your thoughts and emotions flood your bloodstream with cortisol and adrenaline, and your body deals with this as a threat. You may feel as if you are constantly under attack.

When your body does encounter a real threat, such as being chased by a vicious dog, the hypothalamus, a tiny region in your brain, sets off an alarm in your body. The body is wise, and the alarm prompts your adrenal glands, located atop your kidneys, to release a surge of hormones, including cortisol and adrenaline. The stress hormone adrenaline increases your heart rate, elevates your blood pressure, and boosts energy supplies. The primary stress hormone cortisol increases sugar (glucose) in the bloodstream.

This response of "fight or flight" fuels you to deal with the threat. Your body is meant to return to a normal state once the threat disappears. When stress is constantly present, you feel under attack and the flight or fight reaction stays turned on. This alters immune system responses, damages your health, and impairs your relationships.

This complex alarm system communicates with the area in the brain that controls mood, fear, and motivation. The continuous activation of the stress hormone system, and overexposure to stress hormones, disrupt almost all your body's processes. Anxiety, depression, weight gain, and digestive problems are increased, and they can prevent you from trusting in your body's natural ability to give birth.

Since pregnant women can begin to doubt the wisdom of the body, let's talk about your amazing uterus. The uterus contains two important types of muscles. The circular muscles contract, keeping the cervix closed during pregnancy. These circular muscles must relax to allow the longitudinal muscles to contract during labor. The contractions of the longitudinal muscles enable the cervix to open for the baby to move down through the birth canal. During a fight or flight response, adrenaline causes the circular muscles on the cervix to contract and tighten to prevent further dilation. This is your pregnant body's natural response to keep the baby safe while allowing you to escape!

I hope that this is sufficient for you to understand how important it is to become intimately acquainted with your pregnant body and allow it to feel safe and relaxed.

Your safety is important and medical intervention saves lives in the labor ward. While the technology and observation on a birthing mom is comforting, remember that childbirth is a normal physiological process. It is unfair to assume that your body might fail or, on the other hand, that technology can prevent the reality that complications do arise. Instead of worrying about what can go wrong, rather imagine and plan for things to go right. While you do need gentleness and care, you will find safety in trusting your body's abilities. You are not incapacitated, and most women achieve a normal birth without requesting unnecessary intervention.

Dealing with the Changes

There are many things to change if you are terrified because your life has been precisely planned, your schedules are fixed in fifteen-minute slots, and your personal needs are at the bottom of your priority list. Most people are concerned about how the changes related to pregnancy are going to impact their lives. If this pregnancy is not something you planned, it is still a change to your situation and it is going to require adjustments.

Stressful experiences are a fact of life, and traumatic experiences can stick like barnacles to the bottom of a boat. They are carried around with you. Resistance may seem essential to your survival, but it is actually only the byproduct of inflexibility. If there is no desire to change, you could hide your fears and anxieties by faking an appearance of confidence. To avoid uncomfortable feelings, you could engage in some activity that is usually not dominated by your concerns, fears, or anxiety. It may provide a temporary relief, but soon your concerned thoughts will ricochet and creep back into your mind. Blocking out or resisting change is as hard as swimming against strong invisible ocean currents. However, when you accept that something has to change, it is similar to releasing a drop of ink into water, slowly beginning to color your whole life.

You may not be able to change your current situation in a major way immediately, but you can take steps to manage the impact it is having on you. You will eventually have to stop doing the things that have never worked for you. Identifying what your stresses are, and learning how to reclaim the strength and the wisdom of your body, can help you react to stress in a healthy manner. Your fears become insignificant as your inner world begins to flourish. You will become more comfortable under your skin as you begin to experience an improved quality of life.

Epigenetic & You

Epigenetics is the study of heritable changes. Scientists have determined that events impacting us throughout our lives can influence how our cells interpret genetic material. These influential changes can be passed on to our offspring and possibly into future generations. If a mother is stressed during pregnancy, she will be flooding her system with cortisol and adrenaline. This can impact the regulatory system of an unborn baby, and it can continue into adulthood and affect the child's ability to manage emotions. Other harmful experiences such as malnutrition, exposure to chemical toxins, or use of drugs before birth, are also built into the architecture of the developing brain through the epigenome.

Giving any attention to your circumstances may seem overwhelming, but it is really an opportunity to face challenges with a willingness to heal and bring relief, peace, justice, and love to your heart. Avoidance and denial perpetuate historical patterns in your life. Small steps contribute to overall continuous improvement, and this makes you become inwardly secure.

As your anxiety and stress levels reduce, you will feel calm and your child will feel safe. Supportive environments and relationships generate lower stress maternal surroundings, while adding constructive epigenetic value that activates positive genetic potential in the developing brain. This is the power of making small changes and you are responsible for this.

Bonding with Baby

Your baby is growing physically, and nurturing the emotional connection is equally important as managing the external environment. We know that babies can hear and they can, and do, respond to touch stimuli from outside the womb, especially from the mother. A mother who rubs her belly, and sings and speaks to her unborn child, will convey a sense of love to her baby. The emotional well-being of your unborn child is important, and your pregnancy is the opportune time to strengthen the emotional bond.

Here are a few suggestions on **how to bond with your unborn child**:

1. Play **relaxing or calming music** to your baby.
2. **Relax**—Take a walk, have a warm bath, spend time doing something that makes you happy. Evidence shows that the health outcome for the baby is better when mom is relaxed.
3. Gently **rub and touch your belly**.
4. **Sing and talk to your baby,** knowing that you can be heard. Babies can remember certain sounds and they will be soothed by your voice.

The most valuable thing you can do for yourself is make your life a safe haven. Metaphorically, you are preparing for a marathon. Your body and mind must feel safe and align to your new way of being. It is a good time to relax and to reflect on your habits, behavior, patterns, and explore the relationship you have with yourself. By that I mean you are returning to be more you.

Parents are the bridge between the baby and the world, and it's time to go beyond your limitations and adapt for the shape your life is taking. You are destined to meet yourself closely through the intensity of this journey. There is much to learn and understand about how you interact with yourself and others during this time. What you give your time and energy to certainly defines your experience. Embrace the longing to find and understand the depths of your capacity to be a great parent. You must keep working towards creating a firm foundation within yourself to offer your child the space of a loving home from within.

3

Riley's Story

It is remarkable to consider what you can do in nine minutes. You can make a meal, or win a race, fluctuate through a range of emotions, and make a decision that changes your world and your life. Something can equally change in a brief moment. It shapes your destiny. In nine months, your life can take on a whole new direction as a new developing being inhabits your belly, changing the way you communicate with and see the world.

My friend Riley is a remarkable woman. Riley bought a telescope while she was trying to get pregnant with her first child. "I believe in the creative power of imagination and visualization," she said. She wanted to explore the universe and hopefully discover the magical galaxy her child was travelling from. She imagined him in an alternate galaxy, bursting with energy, about to leap into her belly. Watching seas of constellations nightly filled her with a reverence for energy much larger than herself. Riley felt the opening of an invisible, seamless, sacred, and spiritual connection between her and the stars. She marvelled at the patterns, changing lights, and every twinkle that made her realize how alive and loud everything in the universe is. She felt part of a bigger picture, one that is fast-moving, ever evolving, and creatively intriguing. In the silence, she heard a perfectly wise voice speaking from deep within herself assuring her that everything was going to be fine.

The warm presence inside Riley brought awareness that her purpose in the world had changed. She always wanted to be a mother. Having actively participated in the creation of this new life filled her heart with gratitude. Riley said, "Staring at the great wonder of a starlit sky made me contemplate that babies are born beautiful, playful, curious, fascinated, spontaneous, and unconcerned about anything that the world will eventually project on them. The world is still a perfect place. Babies are more capable of being in the moment—sleeping, feeding, smiling, and crying. Babies are not worried about what happened yesterday, nor are they thinking ahead to plan a future. They are not aware of any danger and there is nothing to be ashamed about. That world begins to change as a baby explores, and we begin to fill their world with our ideas. Often we are wrapped up in our own perceptions that are not necessarily true. At the insistence of this truth, I felt committed to focus on my well-being during pregnancy. I prayed fervently that I would be brave like the other women who did this before me. We will never fully comprehend or make sense of everything that happens to us."

As they waited for months before there was confirmation of their pregnancy, she once assured her husband Max, "This not a test of your manhood. I know what it feels like to want something. When you are waiting for some important news, the world can be obscured by your thoughts and you can start feeling fragile."

Likewise her husband sensed when she doubted her abilities. "Max's nurturing presence always steers me in the right direction. His deep eyes are far-seeing, and he always finds ways to connect me back to my own familiar world. Recently while tending to our garden, he reminded me that 'the fetus and baby to come is like all new life.' Pointing to the seeds in his palm he continued, 'These seeds are flawlessly crafted with all the instructions to swell out of the earth and grow into plants. Inside an acorn an intelligent life force is creating a giant oak tree with all the resources to successfully create a forest. This is the creative power of all living things.'"

Small events and occurrences have the possibility of being amplified and expanded as they ripple into your life with the immortal pattern of all living things. There are endless accounts from both men and women who have undertaken this voyage of pregnancy and childbirth, attesting to its transformative nature. The experience reverberates in an immeasurable and profound way across all areas of one's life. Time is of no significance when it comes to manifesting our deepest desires. Once you have planted the seed of your desires, nurture them with a kind, caring, and tolerant attitude towards yourself.

Max's love for nature in essence aligns him to its profound wisdom and capacity as a creative force that exists in all of life. Riley said, "Sometimes I felt myself glowing in this remarkable, beautiful experience, and other times when I was terrified, he assured me that it was part of the natural progression and fluctuations of motherhood. Max's enthusiasm is contagious, and he is an inspiring coach in my life—my strong, solid, and durable safe place. He reunites my spirit with hope, strength, and confidence. I am thankful to Max."

When Riley discovered that the precise process of how labor is initiated is still being explored, she decided to trust those tiny hands in her belly that carried the infinite gift of life.

Baby, Mom & Labor

We understand that labor is a complex multifaceted process involving hormonal responses from the baby's brain, the mother's brain, and the placenta. The baby has the key role in determining when labor will start, guiding the mother from a hormonal and mechanical perspective.

The high levels of progesterone during pregnancy prevent the uterus from contracting. Towards the end of pregnancy, the level of estrogen increases. It is believed that as the baby produces increased levels of oxytocin, it could be a trigger to the maternal brain to increase estrogen production. This process leads to further oxytocin receptors on the surface of the uterus, increasing the sensitivity to the hormone and the ability to act on it. During the last few weeks of normal term, there is also an increase in prostaglandin to soften the cervix, allowing it to become more responsive to the mechanical process of labor. Prostaglandin also has a softening effect on the pelvic ligaments and, together with relaxin, enable the pelvis to open more effectively during labor.

During the latter part of pregnancy, the baby descends into the pelvis. This is commonly referred to as *lightening*. The presenting part of the baby begins to apply pressure on the internal section of the cervix. When evenly applied, this pressure cascades a trigger reaction that signals the mother's brain to release increased levels of oxytocin. This stimulates contractions that move down over the uterus. The pressure from these contractions causes the baby's head to become more flexed. This is known as *fetal axis pressure*. The pressure assists the baby to descend even lower, also applying greater pressure on the cervix and thereby increasing the amount of oxytocin released in a continuous feedback mechanism.

The primordial dance intensifies between mother and child during childbirth as the baby and the maternal body collaborate with precision in the process. As the baby progresses down the birth canal, it must move into the right position to negotiate the shape of the maternal pelvis. This miraculous feat is known as the *cardinal movement*. When we begin to consider how exquisitely the body performs during childbirth, we are more likely to consider a realistic approach towards labor and make responsible choices. Labor should be approached with the deep respect that it deserves.

I was also increasingly curious during pregnancy. But while furiously looking up the endless information that is freely available about childbirth and parenting, I realized the danger of simply gathering information. You may feel as though you know everything. This prevents you from learning anything new, gaining a new perspective. Solely gathering information is a distraction. It was not my responsibility to only gather information, but rather to become knowledgeable on my options and focus instead on what I wanted to achieve. I was lucky enough to identify this earlier and directed my energy into pursuing it.

Reflection

The presence of new life is shaping the dawn of your new journey. May you find yourself engaged in the pages ahead, and may your life grow meaningful and rich with purpose. I am not a doctor, but I can say that rooted in love and honesty you can explore your options in this mysterious and magical world like it's an adventure. If you were to consider the next nine months a map, then you may want to consider the route and how you will get to term. Whether you make a conscious choice or not to follow your destiny, your destiny will follow you. I would say it is far more dangerous to pretend, to forget and ignore yourself by allowing someone else to make choices for you. You could spend hours just hoping, hurting, longing, thinking, or you can actively work on ideas that give you hope and show you how to cope. You can learn about yourself and understand what best works for you. Consider the idea that small changes create a significantly different final outcome.

4

An Amazing Transformation

Your Encounter with the Invisible—The 1st Trimester (1st 12 Weeks)

You know, with certainty, that you are pregnant. In the first six weeks your baby is referred to as an embryo, following which it is called a fetus. In the first trimester, your baby grows faster than at any other time. You may not look pregnant during this period, but chances are you're definitely feeling it! You start to experience some of the symptoms below.

Symptoms & Suggested Natural Treatments

Morning sickness—Drink ginger Tea. Steep crushed ginger root in hot water. Stay hydrated.

Fatigue—Increased level of progesterone acts as a natural sedative. Rest whenever you can.

Increased urination—The amount of blood increases during pregnancy, and the kidneys process the extra fluid that ends up in your bladder.

Constipation—Increased levels of progesterone can slow the movement of food through your digestive system causing constipation. Iron supplements may also add to this. Include plenty of fiber in your diet. Keep well hydrated.

Heartburn—Pregnancy hormones relax the valve between the stomach and esophagus, and this causes stomach acid to leak into this muscular tube. The result: heartburn.

1. Eat small meals.
2. Avoid sugary and greasy food.
3. Avoid triggers—food and smells that make you feel sick

Note: Acupuncture can provide effective treatment of nausea, constipation, hemorrhoid discomfort, heartburn, and back pain.

Growth—The 2nd Trimester (from Week 13 to Week 27)

Your growing baby is very real, and you should be feeling much better than in the first trimester when the body is adjusting to the pregnancy. At the same time, your baby is not big enough to make you feel uncomfortable.

Symptoms & Suggested Natural Treatments

Braxton Hicks contractions—You might experience these mild irregular contractions as tightness in your abdomen in the afternoon or evening. They are part of the body's preparation for labor.

Skin changes—Skin changes are common, and this usually fades away after delivery. Hormonal changes stimulate an increase in pigment bearing cells (melanin) in your skin. You may notice brown patches on your face, known as *melasma*. A dark line may also be visible down your abdomen. This is known as *Linea Nigra*.

Leg cramps—To prevent leg cramps, stretch your calf muscles before bed. Wear comfortable shoes, stay physically active, and avoid standing for long periods of time. A hot shower or bath or ice massage can provide some relief. For an ice massage, wrap up a large ice block or some ice cubes to make an ice pack, and rub the affected area. With an ice massage, you will experience different sensations—intense cold, followed by burning, aching, and finally mild numbness. At that point, stop. Allow at least sixty minutes between each massage to enable the superficial skin temperature to return to normal.

Notes: Please consult your doctor for other common pregnancy ailments—e.g., urinary tract infections and vaginal discharges. Emotionally, you should feel more up to the challenge of preparing for your baby.

The Countdown—The 3rd Trimester (from Week 28 until Birth)

Your baby's movements are more obvious. A growing baby's size and position may make it challenging for you to feel physically and emotionally comfortable. Rest, take a holiday if you can.

Symptoms & Suggested Natural Treatments

Backaches—Pregnancy hormones relax the connective tissues that hold your bones in place. These changes result in discomfort. Get regular exercise, and sit on a chair with good back support.

Braxton Hicks contractions—These contractions tend to occur more often and become more regular as you approach your due date.

Frequent urination—You will feel more pressure on your bladder as your baby moves deeper into your pelvis.

Heartburn—Eat small regular meals. Avoid fatty food and citrus fruit.

5

A Journey Back to Your Own Beginning

Do you feel as comfortable as Riley and Max were about pregnancy? Wherever you are on your journey, let's get to work. You are stronger and much more capable than you think.

A woman's body is wise and naturally designed to conceive and give birth to a baby. Values, beliefs, relationships, spirituality, physical health, and emotional well-being will affect your pregnancy and birth. We learn values from our parents, peers, mentors, and society, and they are also influenced by our choices and decisions. This blend begins to form your conscious constructs of reality throughout your life, with your outer world becoming a reflection of your inner world.

From about the age of three, a sense of self begins to form and you start developing ideas on how to act in order to get a desired response from other people. As you grow more self-aware, you begin to store ideas that bring the desired results and suppress certain emotions as you feel necessary to fit in. Your core belief system is created through a process of logical deductions, and it governs your daily life. Every experience in your life adds to your body of knowledge, and this is stored in the unconscious emotional brain. Even if you forgot how or why you choose your values, every experience is still fundamental to your life. You are also constantly influenced by thoughts that you may not be consciously aware of. We each look at the world through our own eyes, processing and filtering the information through our own value set, emotions, beliefs, and needs. If you feel overweight, unlovable, too thin, unintelligent, insecure, or that you will never make enough money, this is a reflection of your self-image. To change this image requires us to identify the patterns we follow to keep perpetuating these negative feelings towards ourselves.

We all have the same inner resources. By that, I mean none of us have been excluded from having beautiful human qualities within—generosity, kindness, compassion, confidence, creativity, will power, openness, and honesty. We all have the capacity to change. Each step of your pregnancy journey should be approached with humility and honesty to expand the relationship you have with yourself. Whatever you give your attention to grows, and that means working and honoring all aspects of yourself from the inside out. By making one intentional choice, you can shift your limitations to step out of your comfort zone and begin to experience your expansive nature. This is possible as you open up honestly to yourself, with a willingness to reflect on the turbulence you feel within.

Can you imagine taking charge of how you spend your energy? In the process of rediscovering yourself, you are releasing old patterns and habits to create more room for a better life for you and your new baby. Only you know what it is like to be you, and this makes you the only expert on your life. Fear simply drowns out the whispers in your heart that know the truth, and know what you should do. To become comfortable in your own skin is to be brave enough to listen to what your heart has to say.

Let's go back in time and talk to your inner child to uncover and release the old and untrue. Once you uncover some of your thought patterns, you will begin to see how they lead to certain feelings and behavior. Just reading through some of the forthcoming questions may evoke a sensation, feeling, or image. Answering the questions honestly will help you understand how this affects your day-to-day life.

You & Your Parents

To become the parents we would aspire to be, we must first make peace with our inner wounds. Part of this is breaking down the intergenerational patterns of wounding (including the relationship between us and our parents) that no longer serve us and that we do not want to pass on to our children.

Perhaps we have all been wounded in some way as the result of certain internal beliefs we formed from past actions and words of our parents, friends, family, teachers, and those that we have trusted with our dear hearts. There may be people you look to avoid. People who consider you to be a disappointment, crazy, or irresponsible. These people generally fall into a similar category; that is, we look to blame them for a particular negative internal feeling. Well, the truth is that the past is likely to repeat itself by the choices we make, as long as internal beliefs dominate our thinking and reactions. Meanwhile, your thoughts only have an effect on you. They destroy your ability to trust and they therefore interfere with relationships. It does not matter how far you may have travelled from past traumatic experiences; the associated feelings will re-emerge and perpetuate until released. Here you are free to realize that you do not have to dwell on what was. Your words have the ability to convey your deepest pain and release repressed energy, aligning you more towards your authentic self.

Some of us will openly admit to disappointment, resentment, and frustration towards our own parents. Over their anger, neglect, lack of parental approval and understanding. Feelings of being ignored or controlled and unloved. These feelings are common, straining the relationship between parent and child, leading to feelings of deep sadness and bewilderment. Maybe your parents were incapable of giving you the emotional support that they did not also have. It is not possible for you to offer something that you do not have yourself. You may eventually project any unhealed wounds on your child unless resolved and learned. People who have been abused as children or experienced violence are particularly vulnerable to stress. You were born into that world, and you have survived in it, but you don't have to stay in it. Amazingly, some of the seemingly friendliest and kindest people, often surrounded by many other people, still don't feel truly loved and accepted.

Children are brutally honest. Your child may eventually articulate unknown qualities and aspects of yourself that could inspire or deflate you. It is a good time to reconsider how you can break this cycle by doing things you have never done. This is a safe space to understand, forgive, and accept instead of loathing and reacting to what has happened in the past. Your learning curve will shorten as you improve your openness to listening and restore respect to yourself and others.

In the process of healing your wounds, you will heal your relationships and you will open your connection to others.

Exercise
Below is a practical exercise for you to follow. Some ideas have been added for you to elaborate on.

1. To the list below, you may add what you feel is still required or needed in your life. Then read each item aloud and listen to what you have to say.

Love
_____
_____
_____
_____.

Acceptance
_____
_____
_____
_____.

Approval
_____
_____
_____
_____.

Comfort
_____
_____
_____
_____.

Support
_____
_____
_____
_____.

Trust
_____
_____
_____
_____.

2. List the past experiences or situations that still upset you.
a. When did you feel ignored, controlled, unworthy, or unable to fulfill your parents' expectations?
_____
_____
_____
_____.

b. Who do you associate these feelings with or where did they originate?
_____
_____
_____
_____.

c. How do you react when you experience the above feelings?
_____
_____
_____
_____.

3. Let your hurt, pain, and aches speak. Let them be as petty and as judgmental as you feel.

_____
_____

A POCKET GUIDE TO YOUR PREGNANCY

_____
_____.

4. Have you considered why your parents behaved in this manner?

_____
_____
_____
_____.

5. Were your parents absent?
(Alcohol, drugs, neglectfully working away from home, mental health challenges, divorced or separated, living elsewhere. Companionship, touch, play, closeness, and togetherness are as necessary as food, water, and shelter).

_____
_____
_____
_____.

6. Do you have fond memories of endearing behaviors like rubbing noses, giggling, high-fiving. Other parents cook, bake, or buy gifts. How did your parents express their affection towards you?

_____
_____
_____
_____.

7. How do you think these experiences may have contributed to your learning or your fears?

_____
_____
_____
_____.

8. Is there anything unforgivable?

_____
_____
_____
_____.

9. Do you want to apologize for something?

_____
_____
_____
_____.

10. What are you grateful for?

_____
_____
_____
_____.

11. How much of what you think about them is true, or is this just your interpretation? Where did these ideas come from?

_____
_____
_____
_____.

12. Close your eyes and listen. What do you still hear? Are you still replaying a conversation? Please write this down.

_____
_____
_____
_____.

13. Do you feel that you are useless, messing up again, or incompetent?

_____
_____
_____
_____.

14. Your emotions might trigger a response. Pause. Breathe in deeply. Notice your surroundings. Examine your interaction with your inner mental world, and consider the difference you want to make to what is around you. If you were unsure about how your internal world affects your external world, you may understand that now. For example, you could be in a luxurious hotel, still feeling angry. Now it is possible to understand how your anger impairs your vision and how you can become blind to the wonderful things around you. The idea is to move

from scarcity to feeling more abundant. Once you recognize the items that you would like to experience more abundantly, you can begin to make changes that lead you down this path.

Mindful meditation can help you sort through and turn off the endless chatter in your mind. You are reconnecting to your body and the sensations of sight, smell, sound, and taste of the present moment that it experiences. You can practice mindfulness by simply breathing in and out, observing the breath and tuning into the environment around you. Mindfulness involves observing your thoughts in a detached manner without judging them. You will soon realize that your thoughts are simply your thoughts. Your thoughts do not have to define or control you. By observing your thoughts in a detached manner, you can disassociate from them and learn how to relax. Once you become aware of some negative thoughts, you can replace them with healthier alternatives.

Mindful Meditation

Mindful meditation is a practice of awareness. It improves your ability to hold your attention on a single point for longer and longer periods of time. Meditation allows your mind to rest in the now.

Daily Practice
Start with five minutes and work your way up to longer timeframes. Find a quiet place where you can sit undisturbed.

1. Get into a comfortable position and close your eyes. At this moment, you have nothing else to focus on. Relax, take a deep breath in through your nose, and slowly exhale through your mouth.
2. Take another three deep breaths into your abdomen. Imagine your muscles are limp, loose, and all your stress and tension is

fading away with each breath out.

3. Feel the presence of your calm center. You are mindfully connecting with your core, the source of your inner strength. This center is always present, and you can respond with calmness and grace from there.

4. You are floating in peace and calmness.

5. Slowly become aware of your surroundings. Notice the smells and sounds all around you. Become mindful of what you sense or feel within. You can simply tune into the sound of your breathing. If you are outside, you may listen to the wind or the song of a bird. Feel the sun on your skin, or if you are at the sea, focus on the sound of the water and the smell of the ocean. Awareness is the recognition that you are a part of a greater reality.

6. If your eyes are closed, you may see swatches of color moving around.

7. If there are hundreds of thoughts running through your mind, acknowledge them, and let them float away.

8. Stay in the present moment for as long as you can, building up to around fifteen minutes.

9. Finish the practice by visualizing feeling safe and free, or something that makes you feel happy. Spend about fifteen minutes immersing yourself in this happy place. Use your senses to explore. Smell, taste, hear, and feel it as if you are really there.

10. When you are ready, end your meditation and spend time relaxing with your eyes closed before you resume any activity.

Working on anything new requires patience and discipline. Organize your schedule to reflect a definite place and time to invest in yourself.

Once you begin to feel safe and accept where you are, you will find the strength to make changes. Keep a daily journal to observe and write down your experiences. Have you noticed anything you have not thought of before? Are you feeling more positive, more confident as you perform this daily *practice*?

Post Meditation Affirmations

Use these affirmations for at least twenty-one to twenty-eight days.

- My imperfections make me unique.
- I am worthy of love.
- I love my body.
- My body deserves respect and care.
- I am love and love is all around me.
- I feel safe.

Write down how you feel after twenty-one days.

Exercise
There must be something you admire about your parents. Try to write down at least three things.

_____
_____
_____
_____
_____.

Learning to Free Yourself

Have you noticed that you are free to create and change any thought you want? Some changes may take longer to process but your freedom is worth the effort.

You are learning to free yourself from the very thoughts that have been the source of your pain. Finding the answers to lingering questions—such as "Why did my parents not love me enough?"—can be leave you feeling unsettled. The process of investigating and finding the answers inside you is a way to resolve any discomfort or tension you experience in a relationship. It removes the distortions and judgements, revealing things we may have taken for granted.

For the caterpillar, there is a complete dissolution within the cocoon, and this is what it feels like to dissolve your pain. When you begin to see root causes and answers, you will quickly learn that self-insight does not come from the outside. I want to assure you that only your efforts can bring the depths of healing that can fill you with confidence and strengthen your ability stand up for yourself.

6

What Are My Values?

Helping You Define What Matters to You

Your values are the things that you truly believe are important to you. As you move through life, your values may change. Your values often determine your choices or decisions. You may feel dissatisfied and unhappy when something does not align with a personal value.

Exercise
Clarify what matters to you as an individual.
From the following list, choose ten personal values that are important to you.
Circle them. Add any others that you can think of, but list ten in total.
Cross out four, and narrow your list down to six values.
Cross out three, to further reduce your list down to your three most important values.
Cross out two more, focusing in on the single value that is most important to you.
Think about this one remaining "core" value.

Write briefly about your choice, including answers to these questions:

a. Why is it so important to you?
_____
_____
_____
_____.

b. How would you feel if other people did not share the value?
_____
_____
_____
_____.

c. What is your opinion of those who do not demonstrate this as a core value?
_____
_____
_____
_____.

d. Would you feel comfortable being around someone who did not share this value?
_____
_____
_____
_____.

e. Could you be friends with someone who didn't share this value?
_____
_____
_____
_____.

Achievement	Fame	Peace
Adventure	Family	Pleasure
Authenticity	Friendships	Ethical
Authority	Fun	Popularity
Autonomy	Gratitude	Positive Attitude
Balance	Growth	Recognition
Beauty	Happiness	Religion
Boldness	Honesty	Reputation
Challenge	Humor	Resilience
Citizenship	Influence	Respect
Community	Inner Harmony	Responsibility
Compassion	Justice	Security
Competency	Kindness	Self-Respect
Contribution	Knowledge	Service
Creativity	Leadership	Spirituality
Curiosity	Learning	Stability
Determination	Love	Status
Empathy	Loyalty	Success
Equality	Meaningful Work	Trustworthiness
Fairness	Openness	Wealth
Faith	Optimism	Wisdom

Understanding & Embracing Your Differences

Understanding your core value clarifies why you make certain decisions. Even if your values as a partnership are not aligned, you may be able to anticipate your partner's decisions and learn to eliminate ambiguity. When it comes to making major decisions, understanding your differences creates an opportunity to prevent frustrations or friction, reduces conflict and misunderstandings, and allows you to reach a suitable compromise. This is why we take turns in conversation—listening and sharing, connecting instead of correcting. In this way, differences can become an opportunity to extend your ever-expanding learning base, and they transform into a positive force in your life as you reflect, respect, and accept them.

If you have recently moved to another country or community, you may be aware that the values there are different than your own. It may even be a challenge to maintain your own values while trying to respect theirs. Later you may want to consider the challenges children are faced with as they deal with similar conflicting demands: what parents expect from them and what their peers expect. Most parents have one thing in common; they want the best for their children. If you are reading this book and looking for a deeper understanding, you are definitely one of these, and I am sure that you will allow your child to balance their own identity with how they interact and "fit in" with others.

7

Inspiring New Thoughts

Stage 1: Let's Talk about Your Experience

Everything we say and think creates our experiences. Experience refers to the process of feeling, sensing, and perceiving the world around us and then how we respond to it. Our thoughts are the building blocks used to create our life. Feelings are formed internally and we express them externally in a verbal or nonverbal way. Each thought has a unique structure, and cumulatively, they mirror into the spoken and body language we use.

The subconscious mind does not judge this overall process of feelings translated into a response. Rather, it is the conscious mind and brain that process information from our experiences and the emotions attached to them. Most people cannot count the number of times that they feel they have made a mistake or said the wrong thing. That internal voice reminds them that they could have done better. The voice never keeps count but always drives us to improve. It makes us work harder, and no matter how hard you work, it is still there to remind you to do more.

The subconscious believes what we have to say, negatively or positively, about ourselves, regardless of whether it is true or not. You are experiencing a presentation of the world around you, according to your own perceptions. You are the storyteller of your experiences. You can start redirecting your experience by noticing what positively stimulates your story and internal dialogue each day.

Stage 2: Stimulating Your Internal Dialogue

Self-talk is centered on the way you see yourself. These thoughts are there to remind you of what you should or shouldn't have said, or what you did or did not do. The anxiety of what should have been can often dominate your mind. You may be concerned about how your life is going to change as a partnered parent. You may be concerned about how you are going to juggle your time as a single parent. Maybe you have everything you ever longed for but you still feel unsure about yourself. I know working single parents are concerned about the lack of sleep and how they might have to shuffle around trying to get to work. I understand your concerns around your looks, and if you'll still feel beautiful in baggy pants with an elastic waistline.

Your thoughts are not accurate if they distract you in any way that allows you to forget about how talented, smart, and fortunate you are. Words are powerful, and any negative self-talk is dangerous. It harmfully affects your mood, behavior, habits, and relationships. Any self-defeating talk causes an inner disturbance by bringing up your perceived flaws, all to remind you that you are not good enough until you do better and more.

These thoughts are persistently at play in the background to dismantle your confidence and to remind you to expect the worst. But there is a way to defeat your uncertainties: extract what you have gained from an experience, rather than focusing on the experience itself. For example, you might have encountered situations in your childhood that have made you feel unwanted or like the black sheep of the family. Reflecting on and examining the details of these situations from a less biased perspective can bring a new understanding. Seeing situations from a new light of more self-empathy will lead to growth and wisdom, removing feelings of uncertainty. You can, on your own, make a difference to yourself. The future exists only in your imagination, and it is ready to be built to your liking. Let's take a view of how you perceive yourself by simply looking at your actions and beliefs.

1. List five beautiful things about yourself.

_____
_____
_____
_____.

2. On a bad day, what are your thoughts about yourself?

_____
_____
_____
_____.

3. Have you noticed any differences in the thoughts around yourself?

_____
_____
_____
_____.

4. Only you are aware of your own indecision. Are you constantly arguing with yourself about why you should or should not do something? What decision do you have to make?

_____
_____
_____

_____.

5. Listen to the voice within. Does the decision feel right for you? What do you have to risk? What will happen if you make a decision?
_____
_____
_____

_____.

6. What will happen if you do not make the decision?
_____
_____
_____

_____.

7. Can you see how indecision interferes and limits achieving some changes?
_____
_____
_____

_____.

8. Do you feel safe? Keep in mind that you cannot avoid or control life.
_____
_____
_____

_____.

9. Think about any mistakes you may have recently made and write them down. Did it worry you? What are you worried about now?
_____
_____

_____
_____.

10. Do you feel there are any rules or traditions that do not fit in with your lifestyle? What rules or traditions would you have to break within you to feel free?
_____
_____
_____.

11. How do you feel about your body? Are you comfortable or anxious about the way you look?
_____
_____
_____.

Stage 3: Taking Charge

Once we identify our self-talk, we are able to refocus and strengthen this inner conversation to realign ourselves with our goals. There is no failure if we look beyond the history of our personal experiences. There may be setbacks and outcomes from the choices we make. Yet there is also understanding and acceptance. We learn rapidly by making a choice.

Most people cannot see outside their own beliefs. Worry is simply a painful preoccupation based only on a hypothetical outcome. Many factors affect the transmission of pain: anger, worry, helplessness, fear, anxiety, and depression. You deserve clarity. Work towards becoming aware of how your schedule dictates your thoughts, emotions, environment, and the general way you live your life. We take time to physically maintain ourselves and eat healthily, but often we do very little towards improving our mindset. When we become aware of our choices, we can all take steps to reduce the stress in our lives.

Most people have a tendency to follow a familiar routine but this may simply perpetuate an ongoing cycle. There will always be days that do not go your way but hold on to the thought that you are worthy and lovable. People around you will begin to relax and move towards supporting you. You are deliberately working to rewire your brain. An old neurologist adage follows the principle of "what fires together wires together." This means that the more you run a neural-circuit in your brain, the stronger that circuit becomes.

Put simply, practice makes perfect. Do what makes you feel happy and inspired; it will make achieving your goals much easier. Succeeding feels good! Learning through our experiences also boosts our confidence. Start with a small seed step, and the idea will transform into an illustration of life that continues to grow bigger and brighter, defining all that is possible.

We become less dependent on the outer world when we take responsibility for our own thoughts and actions. There is a wonderful sense of freedom when you know that your life is in your hands, and always has been!

1. List items you wish to experience more of in your life:

    Freedom_____

    Flexibility_____

Spending time outdoors _____

Spending time with loved ones _____

What can you do to feel happier and healthier?
_____
_____
_____.

2. With reference to the items listed in Question 1, what is the least number of steps that can be done to make your life more enjoyable?
_____
_____
_____.

3. What adjustments can you make to achieve these items?
_____
_____
_____.

Three important mindsets help move us closer to achieving our goals:

1. Thoughts create your life every moment of the day.

2. Have a clear vision of the result or dream scenario. Think positively towards it and believe you deserve it.

3. To go from dream to realization, you must take inspired action.

Let's Set an Important Goal

1. Think of something you would really like to achieve and write it down.
   _____
   _____
   _____.

2. When would you like to achieve this goal?
   _____
   _____
   _____.

3. Close your eyes and create a successful image of achieving the goal in your mind.

4. Using your imagination, visualize floating up into the air and moving forward in time until you land above the future date set in your goal. See all the events leading up to your goal. Change and realign them to support your goal. Fully sense how you would feel once this goal has been achieved.

5. Still using your imagination, visualize moving halfway back to the present time. Looking back at your current self, notice what steps you could do now to achieve your goal.

Take action! Start working through each step you visualized. Choose the steps that make you happy first. It will help inspire action and get the ball rolling. You can choose to become closer to your heart by dismissing thoughts that do not support you. By doing so, it will become easier to manage and achieve each step, leading to the realization of the goal.

8

Journaling

I find that some people would rather keep things bottled in, as if they are afraid of drawing attention to themselves by talking. The lack of sound when someone is unhappy is deafening, as it pounds its way into the hearts of our relationships like an invisible storm. When withholding, it is easy to start believing that your anger, grief, and unhappiness are bigger than someone else's.

Journaling is a powerful medium of reflective practice. It is a strategy for structuring our approach to self-reflection. It gives us the ability to self-actualize and verbalize our walled emotions in conscious thought. Here we can question our assumptions and expectations, and gracefully explore ourselves. It is an outlet for our creativity, a way to pen our principles and purge the subconscious of self-conflict.

One word, two, three; and we are writing about the monster that previously consumed our thoughts. We feel the emotions and see the black edges of her coat. The shades of possibility become visible as our thoughts take shape, and allow us to examine our own words with purpose. It can be a catalyst to finally put something behind us and move on. An honest recount can bring awareness and insights that can help us evaluate where we are investing energy. Examining our narrative with a new perspective can lead to clarity of goals and intentions, and remove our fears around them.

We are giving some hurtful experiences the attention they deserve. You may even want to keep a little black book journal that you might eventually burn! By writing we can digger deeper to examine our expectations, disappointments, and challenges in an objective nonjudgmental way, opening a path to better parent-infant interaction, self-forgiveness, and healing. All in our own time, and in a solo situation.

When you journal on a daily basis, you begin to chart your progress, get in touch with your emotions, and visualize a way into the future. Journaling is a wonderful tool to plot your way from dreams to realization.

A Framework for Journaling

A basic reflective framework, centered on the Gibbs Reflective Cycle, can be applied to your daily life. Start your reflective practice by structuring your journal as follows:

Description—What happened?

Feelings—How did it make you feel? What are you thinking? How does it make you feel now?

Evaluate—What was the intention of the situation or person?

Analysis—What sense can you make of the situation or person? How does it limit you?

Action—What steps will you take to move on? Don't forget to write about the good stuff too!

9

Affirmations

Affirmations are positive statements expressed in the present tense. Replace thoughts that tear you apart with reflections of gratitude and positive affirmation. Affirmations are a form of self-hypnosis to reprogram your subconscious mind. You must believe that good health or happiness is accessible to anyone, and your outcomes are possible too. Life will always move forward, even if you choose to do nothing. Only you can let you be who you are, and strengthen the connection from deep within. Affirming one's own worthiness, value, and self brings relief and direction to your life.

Repetition of a phrase rewires the brain and rephrases the way you think about yourself or a situation. We are used to controlling so many aspects of our lives that facing any uncertainty can be a challenge. You can prepare for future difficulties by learning new ways to cope and by letting go of everything that you cannot control. Positively changing the way you think about yourself will motivate you to work towards goals more efficiently.

The use of affirmations should become a daily practice during pregnancy. Create a vision board to bring focus and clarity to what you want to see. Be definite about what you want (intention), and go after it with all your heart (desire). Without a plan, you have no path to your goals.

Success is the miraculous unfolding of our desire into an accomplished goal. Consistency and dedication of practice will improve the way you feel about yourself, and will make you more productive a greater amount of the time. There is deep connection between mind, body, and spirit during childbirth. The transformative journey into motherhood challenges your confidence, strength, and perceptions about yourself and your relationships.

Be clear about what you want in your affirmations. When your mind is unfocused, it tends to jump from one thought to another. The brain requires specific information to work with, and the subconscious mind needs direction. The brain is a powerful mechanism to recognize patterns and we learn by repetition.

By shifting a limiting belief, your world expands with a wider range of options and possibilities. Challenges are seen as opportunities. You will feel less resistant and find solutions to items placed in the "Can't do" or "Unsure" boxes. The responsibility is where it always belongs—in your own hands. Choose an affirmation, and use it as many times a day until you embody the idea.

After twenty-one days, an internal barrier will seem to shift and a new way of feeling about yourself will begin to set in. Give yourself at least twenty-one to twenty-eight days before you move onto another set of affirmations. You are experiencing the wonders of the human body and how it can adapt to create and also shape life.

As this technique of affirmations develops into an ingrained habit after several weeks of practice, it will become easier to use during times of pain and stress.

Exercise

Choose an affirmation that resonates with you from the list below, and add others as your practice develops:

I love and accept myself.

I am supported.

I am naturally successful.

I trust myself.

I believe in myself.

I am strong and deeply connected to my body and baby.

I am amazing and powerful.

Every surge brings me closer to my baby.

I am radiant and confident.

I relax and my muscles relax.

I surrender to my muscles and work in harmony with them for a smooth birth.

I am safe and calm.

My body knows exactly what to do all by itself.

I am surrounded by the love and support of my caregivers.

Life is precious.

I treasure each and every day.

I deserve to be happy.

I choose to take good care of myself.

I sleep easily and peacefully all through the night.

I love eating healthy.

I love my body.

I am radiant and healthy.

I feel energized and enthusiastic.

I am confident.

I am smiling more.

I am a powerful creator.

I expect only the best to happen.

I accept the things I cannot change.

My mind is peaceful and clear.

I appreciate all that I have.

10

Relaxation

Relaxation encourages effective breathing and an increase in your endorphin levels. Endorphins are the body's natural pain-relieving hormones. Relaxation also increases oxygen supply to the body, helping to alleviate both fear and tension which deepen your perception of pain. Using relaxation techniques calms the mother, improving the efficiency of contractions and also speeding up labor.

We can set the tone to relax and let go of everything that no longer positively serves us. By relaxing, you will be able to create a calm, beautiful, and confident place in your mind where you feel safe.

Visualization Technique for Relaxation

I often use a visualization technique in which I imagine myself basking in a golden light that makes me feel strong, confident, and relaxed. Imagine this shower of light over yourself. See it rapidly moving from the top of your head and covering your whole body in a golden wash of relaxation. Notice how relaxed your head, face, jaws, and neck are becoming. This heightened feeling of relaxation is spreading to your shoulders, arms, hands, and down to your fingertips. It flows through your torso into your hips, thighs, buttocks, and all the way down through your legs, shins, ankles, feet, and to your toes.

Relax. Breathe.

Say, "I believe in myself and I trust my body." Feel the connection to your own inner strength and determination. Know within yourself that you want to achieve the best for you and your baby. Gently close your eyes and picture yourself coping really well. See yourself embracing every contraction. Think of it as a pulsating wave of energy. See every surge of this wave bringing you closer to meeting your beautiful baby. You feel safe, energized, and enthusiastic. You are amazed at how strong and capable you are. You are happy and smiling, holding your baby skin to skin.

Choose to feel good! By focusing on feeling good, you will program your subconscious mind to expect good health and smiles. Feel your body relax. Use this space of feeling happy, healthy, and energized to continually affirm your intention of positive outcomes.

11

Preparations to Be a Great Dad

This is a journey to the center of your heart. Dads, unless you are an experienced paramedic, doctor, or nurse, nothing in life would have prepared you for the experience of childbirth. Be open, and approach this new experience by learning about it. There is an opportunity to become engaged in many aspects of the pregnancy.

Talk about how you can balance your work life, finances, household chores, cooking, and laundry. Discuss a birth plan, and become familiar with ways to support your partner. Talk about all the changes and how you will both work to meet these new expectations. This open approach will keep you engaged and involved, and it will help you to not devalue yourself by feeling guilty or incapable.

When someone is in pain, routine common sense is unlikely to prevail. Work to develop a support system with your partner early in the pregnancy, to give you the best possibility of good outcomes as the term progresses. Feeling prepared and empowered will stop you feeling despondent, or retreating when you are not sure of what to do.

There will be a significant increase in household chores in the near and for the foreseeable future. It is a good time to re-evaluate and discuss some adjustments to make it manageable. You may even want to consider hiring a weekly cleaning service or accepting some help from family and friends. You may want to plan and cook some of your favorite meals for the freezer. Get into the process and rhythm of being prepared. Work towards consciously nourishing your desire to succeed. Anything else that does not align to your success must be released and replaced with thoughts of how you will succeed. Even in the most trying circumstances, Dad you are needed!

Your role has changed, and it is not unusual if you are struggling to adapt or you have fears around meeting certain expectations. I can imagine just thinking about your fears can be challenging or overwhelming. This is your mind simply trying to protect you from something that is unfamiliar. Challenges will always arise. We should always work towards acquiring new ways of coping. Believe in yourself and your abilities; it will help you conquer your fears and allow you to succeed.

A change in perception is often all we need. If you feel that you are carrying too much of a burden, or that the task ahead seems monumental, try shifting and undertaking changes in small positive steps. Seeing your potential and experiencing these small accomplishments will boost your inner strength and confidence.

Self-assurance is settling for both you and your partner, which can lead to better and more positive outcomes.

Exercise

Below is a simple exercise to practice. It is a great way to harness a positive state.

Find a quiet place.

1. Close your eyes, take a few deep breaths. Allow your body to relax. Visualize and draw an imaginary heart and place it in front of you.

2. In your own time, imagine all your good qualities, every goal that you have achieved, and all the good things you have done. Feel the many sources of positivity that reside within you. Feel the beauty of your good deeds. Experience and imagine how wildly successful you felt about your achievements. Visualize and place all of this beautiful imagery into the heart sitting in front of you. Let it fill you with confidence.

3. Whenever you feel uncertain, find a quiet place and take a moment to become still. Imagine yourself looking into the heart for the resources and encouragement needed to make your decision. Feel inspired as you see the heart becoming brighter and bolder. Take all the time you need, knowing that you'll find the resources to make your decisions more spontaneously. In this positive state, you will find strength to become more available, attentive, dependable, and affectionate. This is the process to connect you to your true power—inner strength and self-worth. It will build your self-confidence and allow you to nurture the good qualities of the people in your life. This inner strength and self-assurance make other people feel safe and relaxed in your presence.

Note to Dads: Take paternity leave if you can. Once you leave work or the office, be fully immersed in home life. Your partner might be looking forward to some adult company, someone who will simply listen to what they have to say. As you work together as a team, magic happens—your love and feelings for one another will deepen.

Affirmations for Dads

The use of positive affirmations will help to recondition your mind and focus it on the healthier aspects of life. Turn inward to free yourself from emotions that no longer serve you. Be clear about what you want in your affirmations. When your mind is unfocused, it tends to jump from one thought to another. The brain requires specific information to work with, and the subconscious mind needs direction.

The brain is a powerful mechanism to recognize patterns, and we learn by repetition. By shifting a limiting belief, your world expands with a wider range of options and possibilities. Challenges are seen as opportunities. You will feel less resistant and find solutions to items placed in the "Can't do" or "Unsure" boxes.

The responsibility is where it always belongs—in your own hands. Choose an affirmation and use it as many times a day until you embody the idea. After twenty-one days, an internal barrier will seem to shift, and a new way of feeling about yourself will begin to set in. Give yourself at least twenty-one to twenty-eight days before you move onto another set of affirmations.

I am a great dad.

I am worthy of love.

I get better at being a father every day.

I am healthy and full of energy.

I love and respect my partner (name) and child (name).

I am strong and confident.

I trust myself.

I am enough.

I love and respect myself.

LUCY BEAR

I am open to new opportunities and possibilities.

I am in a loving relationship.

I enjoy being with my baby.

I release all fear and worry.

I am enjoying a healthy life.

Money flows to me.

I am supported.

12

Making Changes as a Couple

One part of you may prefer you and your relationship to continue unchanged, while the other part is already aware that changes are underway. Both partners in a relationship rarely have the same feelings and viewpoints across all perspectives of parenting. We are all different and we need to accept this. We often create expectations, only to feel let down and disappointed when they are not fulfilled.

Be empathetic, place yourself in your partner's shoes, and learn to see from their perspective. We can learn to understand that cultural values and beliefs influence how people act. You are not responsible for convincing someone else that they need to improve or change aspects of themself. By creating harmony and balance, you can grow the contents of your relationship. Think of what you would like to enjoy more of, and how you can contribute to achieving this within the relationship. Tell the truth, and nothing but the truth. It will equip you to see life in a new way. It will also nourish a deeper relationship from within.

We are constantly looking for happiness and a way to feel complete. Wholeness is possible for all of us, as individuals. Everything you have ever desired is within you, and accessible to you, as soon as you decide. True happiness is rooted in self, and if you are looking for a person to provide this feeling, then look into the mirror. Make your life more enjoyable by building the foundations of happy and healthy values, beliefs, and attitudes towards yourself. Your sole obligation is to accept that you are worthy and deserving of true love and companionship, and that it will nourish your existence. Once you have established these firm roots within, you will be able to make changes as a couple.

Exercise

Complete the exercise below to form a list of behaviors or situations you would like to improve. Be specific around each item. Rank them in the order of importance to you.

My Top 10 List of Behaviors or Situations that I Don't Like
Example: I don't like that you go out with your friend while I am alone at home.

1._____.

2._____.

3._____.

4._____

A POCKET GUIDE TO YOUR PREGNANCY

_____
_____.

5._____
_____
_____.

6._____
_____
_____.

7._____
_____
_____.

8._____
_____
_____.

9._____
_____
_____.

10._____
_____
_____.

Rewrite the list above, this time reframing and restating each point in a positive manner and in the present tense.

Example: I would like to spend more time together.

1. _____
_____
_____
_____.

2. _____
_____
_____
_____.

3. _____
_____
_____
_____.

4. _____
_____
_____
_____.

5. _____
_____
_____
_____.

6. _____
_____
_____
_____.

7._____
_____
_____
_____.

8._____
_____
_____
_____.

9._____
_____
_____
_____.

10._____
_____
_____
_____.

Examine each point again, and think of one step that could be done to start making the change you would like to see.

Example: We can set aside dedicated time at least once a week to spend quality time together.

1._____
_____
_____
_____.

2._____
_____
_____
_____.

3._____
_____
_____
_____.

4._____
_____
_____
_____.

5._____
_____
_____
_____.

6._____
_____
_____
_____.

7._____
_____
_____
_____.

8._____
_____
_____
_____.

9._____
_____
_____
_____.

10._____
_____
_____
_____.

13

Working on Your Relationship

I know it can be difficult to admit, especially to yourself, that you may be uncertain or unhappy in your relationship with your partner. Unhappiness can be experienced in different forms, having lasting impacts on our well-being if left unchecked. If you do feel unhappy, I encourage you to consider the characteristics of your relationship, and implement steps to bring more joy into your life.

A healthy relationship consists of many of the following characteristics and qualities:

1. A choice and commitment by both partners to work on, and improve, the relationship.
2. Partners are attuned to how each think and feel about a situation.
3. Both partners have aligned desires, or they can arrive at a healthy agreement about important matters such as children, finances, careers, and household life.
4. Major decisions are made after mutual consideration.
5. Each partner is considerate, respectful, and understanding of the other's feelings.
6. You feel confident! Your partner feels confident. Both partners are supportive and inspire each other to bravely step into the world.

7. There is trust, commitment, friendship, and respect for each other's individual needs.
8. There is mutual generosity, each giving and sharing.
9. Partners are protective of each other. You feel safe.
10. Each partner agrees that they are individually worthy of love and happiness.
11. Both partners feel grateful to have the other person in their life.

It is time to reconsider the nature of your relationship and examine its characteristics when:

1. You are unable to communicate your feelings. You feel dismissed at any fair attempt to express yourself. You are being constantly criticized. These feelings shrink you, making you feel insecure and destroying your confidence.
2. Your partner's priorities supersede yours. Your partner values only what they want. This uncaring attitude makes you feel disposable and unwanted.
3. You feel frightened. You feel constantly stressed about how something you might say or do is going to upset them. These feelings destabilize you.
4. Your partner is dishonest. A relationship can only grow when it is based on truth.
5. Your partner does not apologize or take ownership of abusive behavior. They may apologize, but make no effort to change this ongoing behavior.
6. Parenthood is unwanted.

The longer you are involved with someone who is toxic, the more you deprive yourself of making a true connection with someone who truly values you. It is exhausting, frustrating, and stifling to give your energy to someone who should not be in your life. Why deprive yourself of the possibility of connecting with someone that matches your level of interest and commitment? We are all worthy of happiness. I feel no joy drifting through life. There is more to life than simply going through the motions of recurring days, with each passing day feeling as empty and uninspired as the previous ones. If your needs are not met, then you are responsible for changing this outcome. This means holding back the unrequited energy you are giving to an unbalanced relationship, and making room to explore changes that will bring you more joy.

Inaction can be viewed as an action, given that it is a *choice* not to address anything. Allowing your own joy to sit in intermission can lead to confusion, shame, guilt, anxiety, unhappiness, and feeling the constant need to be right. But we can unlearn all these habits. We can utilize our experiences from unfavorable circumstances and situations to define a new roadmap of change. It is one thing to *desire* something, but a different step to make a *decision* to go after it. It can be life changing. And it is certainly empowering.

I encourage you to explore the many facets of your relationship. Writing down our feelings helps us to structure our thoughts, which may feel daunting and overbearing when only internalized. Writing can help you identify where you should focus your concerns, and where adjustments have to be made. Be patient as you learn about yourself and your relationship.

Remember that you will have to live with your answers. Responsible choices take into account the consequences. Before you decide to continue to stay in your relationship or end it completely, it is a good idea to take a step back and reflect. Changes might not be fast or easy, but they are usually never as difficult as we initially perceive them to be. Pause. Take time to ensure that you understand the whole story. If you feel a need to steer in a new direction, know that you will likely encounter blind spots, blocks, and resistance that could potentially take you completely off course. But remember that you are resilient, immensely powerful, and you possess all the magnetic qualities to attract a more fulfilling life.

The idea is to focus on what you want to achieve or change, rather than what you fear. Close your eyes for a moment. Feel the power of your imagination and inner strength. Know that you can always use this strength to accelerate change. Follow the direction of your heart and trust your inner desires to steer you onto the right course. You will know that you are on your right path once you begin to overcome the pain and chaos of an unhappy relationship, and begin to replace the experience with progress and growth.

If you feel compelled to stay with someone who does not reciprocate your interest and commitment, then you are part of your own root problem. You deserve clarity, and I propose that you respond honestly and graciously to the questions in the exercise below. I understand how difficult it is to write or even think about a one-sided response, but I encourage you to try. As you start to question what you consider to be reasonable and normal, you will become aware of what needs to change.

Exercise
1. How does your relationship make you feel?
_____
_____
_____
_____.

2. How did your relationship start and why did you enter it?
_____
_____
_____
_____.

3. Has the relationship changed since it started?

_____
_____
_____
_____.

4. Does your partner bring value to the relationship?

_____
_____
_____
_____.

Relationships are a partnership between two people. While the dynamic is centered on a pairing, wholeness and happiness starts with oneself. Consider your own contributions to the relationship as you build your path forward. Both you and your partner should be able to independently, and honestly, answer questions around your relationship. If you both have similar conclusions, and feel the relationship is worth saving, then each person will have to contribute towards creating more joy.

Use the following prompts to discuss ways to improve your relationship with your partner:

1. How did we arrive here?

_____
_____
_____
_____.

2. Can we identify the elements that are not going well?

_____
_____

_____.

3. Do we both agree that the relationship is worth saving?
_____
_____
_____.

4. Are we both willing to invest time, energy, honesty, and effort into building more joy into our relationship?
_____
_____
_____.

5. Can we find new ways to effectively communicate, understand, and share our needs?
_____
_____
_____.

6. Do we need professional help or need to take time apart?
_____
_____
_____.

Emotions dictate your actions, thoughts, and intentions. Try not to react or make decisions that you may regret. Rather determine how you intend to work out a solution that is expansive for you and the best way forward for you, in any scenario. Don't look for perfect solutions.

However, if you feel the relationship cannot be salvaged and is headed for destruction, then you'll need to openly discuss this with your partner. Taking time apart can give you new perspectives, and help see a way forward—be it alone or together. If separating from your partner is the best way forward for you, then you may want to consider some additional external support to help you.

1. Do you have family or a friend that is willing to help you?
_____
_____
_____
_____.

2. Are there any thoughts that get in the way as you consider the changes you want to make?
_____
_____
_____
_____.

3. Are these thoughts reasonable?
_____
_____
_____
_____.

4. How will these changes likely impact you in the short-term?
_____
_____
_____
_____.

5. Can you come up with ways to manage the impact of these short-term changes?
_____
_____
_____
_____.

Think of three steps that you can work on immediately to manage any short-term changes. Give one item priority, and review how you feel in a few days. Each step is intended to bring you closer to the outcome that you desire.

Example: I will manage and plan my finances better. I can make a budget according to my direct needs.

1._____
_____
_____
_____.

2._____
_____
_____
_____.

3._____
_____
_____
_____.

After a few days, revisit the exercise and see if you are ready to tackle the next step or add to your list. Take more time if you need, but remember to follow through on and complete each step. As you begin to heal, you will start responding to each step with more calmness and strength.

14

Visualize Your Dreams and Goals

Athletes use visualization to picture winning or playing the perfect game. We can also use positive language to get into the "zone," and focus in on our goals. Researchers infer that sport performance has more to do with mental ability and strength, rather than physical ability only. If your internal critique interferes, work towards making this voice softer each day until it completely disappears. Visualization activates the creative powers of the subconscious mind, motivating us to seek internal creative solutions. There is a magnetic pull towards your goals as you visualize yourself succeeding. You will notice a change in your motivation, and a desire to do things that you once avoided. Even when athletes are physically and mentally challenged, they have deep mental resources that allow them to remain ambitious, determined, and optimistic.

Exercise

Find a comfortable place to sit undisturbed.

1. Close your eyes. Take a deep breath in through your nose, and exhale slowly through your mouth. Allow yourself to relax.

2. Take another long, slow, deep breath, and hold that breath for a moment. Now exhale, slowly.
3. One more time enjoy another long, slow, deep breath, and let go of all your stress and tension as you exhale.
4. With your stress and tension fading, breathe at your own natural comfortable rate.
5. Feel your muscles relaxing.
6. Picture and feel yourself laughing, smiling, and feeling happy. Experience these emotions attached to your success.
7. Imagine your desired outcome as vividly as possible.
8. Imagine a labor full of love, energy, enthusiasm, and strength.
9. Imagine making a fantastic living while being happy, and immersed in this new life with a baby.
10. Note any thoughts that interfere with your outcome and imagine them drifting away.
11. See that you have all the resources for success: you can feel and use them.
12. See yourself succeeding.

You are undergoing a rehearsal each time you practice this technique. The more you see yourself succeeding, the more confident you will become. Focus on inspiring yourself with a clear vision, and moving towards it.

15

Hypnobirthing

Hypnobirthing is a pain management technique that you can learn and practice in advance. Grantly Dick-Read, a British obstetrician, concluded that women who felt relaxed during labor felt less pain. He devised a "fear-tension-pain cycle" as a way of explaining how emotional responses can increase the intensity of pain. He suggested that fear caused women to become tense, and that the tension increased pain. Our muscles become tense as we prepare for attack or escape during a fear response. This is known as a "fight or flight response." Learning to relax reduces tension, which in turn reduces pain.

Hypnotic language is designed to focus attention and turn it inward. It is a form of deep relaxation. Practicing this exercise frequently will train you to relax during increased levels of tension during birthing. The exercise is best practiced with another person to guide you through each step.

Exercise

You can record the following exercise and play it back. Or if you prefer, there are many similar online exercises. Choose what is comfortable for you.

Find a quiet place, lie down, and relax into a comfortable position.

Close your eyes as you breathe in and out, and allow every muscle in your body to relax.

5..... 4..... 3..... 2..... 1..... 0..... Choose to sink deep down into hypnosis.

Take a deep breath in, breathe out, and let go of everything you don't need.

Relax as you breathe in, deeply and fully.

Slow down your breathing to a gentle, natural rhythm.

Thank each breath for giving you life. Feel the healing power of your breath sweeping through your body.

Thank your body. Rub your hands together and feel your energy.

Say aloud, "I love and appreciate my body."

Feel yourself drifting in love, knowing that this relaxation is benefitting you and your baby.

Focus on these positive suggestions for birth:
"My body knows how to give birth."
"I am confident and my body is powerful."

Focus on your abdomen and lower pelvic area. Allow these muscles to relax.

Release any tension you feel in your abdomen and lower pelvic area. Picture your tension melting away through your feet and into the ground.

Relax. Trust your body to work in perfect harmony with your baby.

Accept *all* sensations... With each breath, you are more and more relaxed, at ease and focused.

To prepare for the birth, repeat the following affirmations:
"I will carry each sensation and trust my body."
"I am nurtured by those around me, quietly encouraging me."
"I am doing an amazing job."
"Women all over the world will be birthing with me."
"I can meet the different energy of transition with courage and acceptance."
"I am doing such a great job."

Breathe down to your belly and to your baby.

Repeat these additional affirmations:
"I am open to all the different rhythms of the birth journey."
"My muscles will naturally fan out and give way to make room for my baby."
"My baby will crown with ease."
"Our baby is welcomed with open arms."

Run through the affirmations again if you want to extend the length of this hypnosis session.
Open your eyes in 5... 4... 3... 2... 1... or drift off to sleep.

16

The Benefits of Organizing Your Family and Friends

Satisfaction, security, and support, are needs that we have an innate desire to fulfill. Experiencing these qualities gives us confidence to reach a desired positive outcome. This is especially true in the process of labor and childbirth. I encourage you to rally family and friends early in your pregnancy, building a team to support you. Support comes in many shapes: it can take the form of emotional reassurance and praise in early term, all the way to progress updates in the midst of labor. We all need people by our side to offer comfort, coping techniques, a warm soothing touch, or even to speak up for us when we are unable to do so. Research has found that continuous support at the time of labor and childbirth leads to an increase in the mother's likelihood of a vaginal birth without adverse effects. Being supported was also seen to encourage a steady release of endorphins, enhancing non-pharmacological pain relief for the mother. These natural measures reduce the need for medical interventions, such as caesarean sections, and synthetic pain relief. A natural vaginal birth is usually safer for both the baby, and the laboring mother. A safer and more positive outcome during childbirth will generally also lead to a more favorable postpartum outcome for baby and mother.

In some cultures, expectant parents are supported by family and friends through, and well after, childbirth. Grandparents, extended family, and friends are actively engaged in the upbringing of children. This village approach has been seen to have long lasting positive effects on children. If you find yourself feeling slightly isolated entering your pregnancy journey, my hope is that you will find a way to start or refresh relationships around you and build your village. It is a good idea to meet with your family and your partner's family, if they plan to be active supporters during your pregnancy and after birth.

Our parents have already faced the challenges of being new parents. Every parent-child relationship is unique, and will have its own nuanced set of interactions and expectations. If you have concerns about your own parents' differing beliefs or choices around childbirth, now is a good time to discuss it with them. Your concerns could be about what happens to the placenta, or around circumcision. The process of when, or how, to the name the baby can be challenging in some traditions. According to the Kabalarian Philosophy, a balanced name that harmonizes with one's date of birth enhances a child's positive qualities, and draws them to their core purpose. Spiritualists may resonate with the idea that naming a baby calls on their soul energy, and activates their unique soul gifts. I am sure that we can all agree that our brain processes information based not only on what we hear, but also the emotions attached to it. In any circumstance, by expressing your baby's name with affection, you are making your child feel wanted and loved.

Astrology, rituals, or traditions have played an important and large role in many cultures. People have followed some of these rituals or traditions for several generations, many not questioning their feelings towards them. Open discussion is essential in organizing and building support that aligns with the outcome *you* desire. The exercise below can be used to help understand family traditions that differ from your current beliefs. Answering the questions alone can be less intimidating than an initial confrontation, and can help you build up towards openly discussing the topics with your family. Even if you do not agree with all traditions, you may want to understand their heritage, or find ways to respect any that are significant to your relatives.

Exercise

1. Why do you think the tradition is important?
_____
_____
_____.

2. What is the intention of your family continuing the tradition?
_____
_____
_____.

3. How would your family feel if you disagreed with their view?
_____
_____
_____.

4. How would you feel if your family disagreed with your view?
_____
_____
_____.

5. Is it worth having an uncomfortable or distant relationship over the differing view?

_____
_____
_____
_____.

6. How can all parties compromise to reach an acceptable situation?
_____
_____
_____
_____.

All relationships should have equal parts of listening and sharing. Be open to listen, even if you do not like what is being said. Share freely; express your own desires or needs. There is a possibility that a differing opinion may in fact only be a different perception. Minimize any unease or conflict by giving your family and friends the attention, and understanding, that you would appreciate receiving when reinforcing your needs. Feeling heard and respected deepens the mutual trust, connection, and support.

There are many adjustments with having a newborn in your home. It can often feel overwhelming. You may want help with the laundry, meals, cleaning, or the care of pets. Establish how you would like to be supported, and then discuss these roles clearly with your family and friends.

Consider a skill or talent that each person in your support group may have, and how they can assist you. Sharing your ideas will ease fears, while helping to build everyone's motivation and understanding of how to support you.

Exercise

1. Make a list of people who are likely to visit you after the baby is born.

_____
_____
_____
_____.

2. Make a list of people whose opinions and assistance you value. List specific items or tasks where you will require help.

_____
_____
_____
_____.

3. Link each specific item or task to an appropriate person in your close support group. Discuss the task with the person and ways to facilitate the assistance.

_____
_____
_____
_____.

As you build deeper relationships with your core supporters, you may also want to consider if your choices are building distance between you and any wider family or friends. Healthy relationships nurture you, reduce stress, and contribute to your well-being. Well-balanced but distant relationships can also be enriching during their occasional exchanges. Even if this idea scares you, imagine that everyone is excited about your newborn. Consider ways you can include some of these people. It could simply be to briefly welcome your baby.

While being around a new baby can be a very exciting time, not everyone is capable of offering you the support or well wishes that you deserve. I encourage you not to spend time with people who exhaust and deflate you. Lack of sleep, pain, feeding, and newborn care are all already tiresome! This is a good time to discuss general guest visitation to your home with your partner or family.

Remember that even after your baby arrives, you will still have your own needs and desires. Sleeping, getting your hair done, sleeping, doing something you enjoy, meditating and sleeping. You need help! Having the right people around you can be wonderful. You will greatly appreciate the extra help, and preparing for this now will make your new life a little easier. Rest and sleep at every opportunity. Your mental and physical well-being can suffer without sleep, and this can lead to depression and anxiety. You are going to need extra calories each day for breastfeeding. It would be fantastic to have family or friends organized to cook hot nutritious meals, take you to follow-up appointments, and to look after the baby while you shower or rest. Planning ensures that you are not overwhelmed by tasks or visitors alike. It also sets out clear roles for people, so not to overburden anyone willing to extend their help.

17

Assert Yourself

Articulating your needs does not have to imply being disrespectful, careless, or inconsiderate with your words. Learn to express your thoughts clearly and politely. You are acting in your best interest, and that is the difference between being assertive and aggressive. Learning to effectively communicate will help you clearly convey a different perspective and foster conflict resolution in all aspects of your life. Finding your voice will empower you to change your worn-out response patterns, and lead to new opportunities of self-fulfilment. It can take time to develop and learn how to effectively express yourself. Keep refining your communication abilities until it feels natural. Be friendly and approachable; your positive attitude and candid words will land on open ears.

18

A Recap

Let us take a moment to reflect on all the work, exercises, and daily practices you have embraced. Well done! I hope you find yourself positively adjusting to your new role as a parent. Were all your fears as real as you thought they were? Were you able to find ways to address all your concerns? Taking small steps forward has been the fundamental path to growing, and ultimately, to your desired successful outcomes. Your viewpoint may have significantly changed as you found ways to dive deep into exploring yourself, and your needs. Many exercises may have challenged some of your long-standing perspectives. Allow yourself time to settle, but keep focused on what you would like to achieve. Remember that you are resilient and resourceful. Take time each day to close your eyes, say your affirmations, and reflect on your new way of thinking. Use affirmations that feel true and comfortable to you. The practice will become part of your daily routine, and begin to redefine your belief system. At this reflection point, we can take the opportunity to work through any of your remaining concerns, while also reframing your outlook and goals.

Exercise

1. Briefly list any concerns, or apprehensions, you may have. These feelings could be rooted around your family, relationships, your baby,

or even with yourself.
_____
_____
_____
__ _____.

2. Acknowledging these feelings may make you feel uncomfortable. Do you feel your body becoming tense? Describe how you feel.
_____
_____
_____
_____.

3. Challenge these feelings.
Why do you believe these feelings to be true?
Have you learnt any practices that you can embrace to resolve these feelings?
_____
_____
_____
_____.

Your Goals

Complete the exercise below to help structure your outlook and goals in a positive frame.
Become aware of your thoughts and emotions, and how they affect your life. Some examples have been included to demonstrate the power of reframing. Working your thoughts and goals into a positive frame strengthens your self-confidence and your ability to achieve goals incrementally.

Negative Frame	Positive Frame
I can't do it.	I can do this. I can achieve anything.
There is no point in trying.	I have inner strength and I am determined.
It is impossible.	I am determined and successful.
I am not good enough or deserving.	I am unique and worthy.
It is too late.	I learn easily. New ideas flow to me.
Identifying my thinking patterns—Thoughts	**Reframing a thought takes away the pressure**
I want things to be perfect.	I am always learning and discovering new things. I can do this my way.

1. What do I value about myself?
_____
_____
_____
_____.

2. Why do I love my life?
_____

_____
_____
_____.

3. What am I grateful for?
_____
_____
_____
_____.

4. What do I like about myself?
_____
_____
_____
_____.

5. Who do I see in the mirror?
_____
_____
_____
_____.

6. What are my goals for this week?
_____
_____
_____
_____.

7. Reflect on your personal and work life. Can you think of any ways to create more time for rest, exercise, fun, and to create healthy meals?
_____
_____
_____

_____.

8. List items and activities that make you feel more relaxed.
Examples: regular massage, music, dance, short walks.

_____
_____
_____

_____.

9. Are you open to trying new experiences? Joining a meditation class or a regular exercise group are both great for your well-being. List any new experiences that you would like to try to help further your feeling of relaxation.

_____
_____
_____

_____.

10. Set your intention—write down what you aspire to achieve. Place no limitations or boundaries on yourself. Spend a few moments to focus on the image of it coming true, and then write it down.

_____
_____
_____

_____.

After completing the exercise, take five minutes to deeply relax. Breathe in fully, and exhale all the way down through your abdomen. Examine your responses to the above exercise. Allow yourself space, and time, to understand ways in which you can resolve any remaining concerns. Honor yourself in the coming week, and commit to undertaking some of the experiences you listed.

19

Your Body Is Changing—Are You Going to Change?

Your growing baby is fed by *placental circulation*, which derives its nutrients from your bloodstream. Your baby receives all its nourishment for growth of nerves, muscles, bones, and organs from this supply. If you have an unhealthy lifestyle and diet, your baby will not have a nutrient-rich source for healthy development during the pregnancy. The metabolic processes that sustain life are complex and interdependent. A well-balanced, nutrient-rich diet will ensure that both you and your baby will have the energy and building blocks for growth, repair, and regulating bodily function.

Eating responsibly means that you are looking for solutions and cultivating eating habits that restore or maintain your vitality. You may want to formulate a flexible and achievable plan that finds a balance between health and indulgence, in order to give your body food that supports it. Eat a wide variety of foods, as close to their natural state as possible. Imagine, for example, that your body performs like an orchestra. You can constantly work to compose and refine the way you eat. Pause for a moment, and observe the ingredients of your meals. Become aware of what you are eating, and when, while refining your choices for better overall health.

If you are stressed, your body is set up for a "fight or flight" response, and it demands more energy. When your body is on stress alert, it becomes efficient at storing its fat. Your body releases fats and produces sugar to fuel your fight or flight. When it comes to willpower versus your survival fight or flight response, the latter is always stronger. If you are dealing with stressful situations throughout your day, it is likely that you may reach for more food than you need. You may also find yourself craving foods that comfort you. Your desire to eat a slice of cake is likely to overcome any idea of settling for an apple! My hope is that you can see the link between your eating habits and anything that is causing a disturbance in your life. Once you understand the underlying causes, it is much easier to work towards a solution.

Do you feel any discomfort or stomachache after a meal? Any unprocessed trauma is stored in your body as cellular memories. Undigested emotions can elicit gut pain. Your body has a messaging system—if you are tired, you need to recognize the need to rest. By paying attention to your body's sensations, you can become aware of the valuable information it contains. Distressing events leave a physical imprint. Your body will store this information until it is consciously released. Living in situations where negative factors are an ongoing threat to your wellbeing—such as divorce, violence, emotional abuse, the loss of significant relationships, and financial difficulty—can all cause emotional distress. While sensations and sounds in your gut are related to what you eat, they are also linked to your thoughts and emotions.

Your earliest nourishment begins in the womb. Emotional and stressful eating may even begin in the womb, as the baby experiences the flow of its mother's energy and emotional state. It is worth resolving and breaking these patterns during this period.

A Few Steps That You Can Take Now

You can reframe your connection to food, and gain more insight, when you look at what goes into your body. What, when, and how you eat has an effect of either supporting or hindering how your body functions. *Eating well has to do with nutrition.* Your cells are made from the food you eat. Once you make an effort to take responsibility for your health and life, you will find practical and effective ways to bring your body into balance.

1. **Eat your meals without being distracted by a TV, or your phone.** Every time a thought distracts you, bring your attention back to the food and its taste. Eat slowly and chew fully before swallowing. You will enjoy your food more and eat significantly less.
2. **Plan your meals.** Make a list of all the items you need to purchase before leaving to the grocer. Having a list will save you time, and encourage you to follow your food plan. Treat your food and meals with respect.

    Ask yourself:

- What will I eat for breakfast?
- What healthy snack will I add to my shopping list?
- What will I eat for lunch?
- What will I eat for dinner?

1. **Prepare your meals in advance.** That way, you can avoid reaching for an unhealthy quick fix. You are taking responsibility for what goes into your body. Adopting moderation of certain food is a better long-term habit than being severely strict.
2. **Keep a daily list of what you eat**; it will help you monitor your habits.

3. Do you feel the need to eat until "My plate is clean"? **Use a small plate.**
4. **Eat smaller, more frequent meals.** Pack healthy snacks—nuts, seed, greens, and fruit.
5. Salt supports many internal biochemical processes in our bodies. **Use unrefined salt or kelp.**
6. **Use natural spices to improve the taste of food.**
7. **Homemade soups are nutrient rich.** Chicken, other red meats and fish contain minerals in a form that the body can easily absorb. Use a variety of bone in your soup base: oxtail, knuckles, marrow bones, shins, and shanks. Animal bones are rich in magnesium, calcium, phosphorus, potassium, natural gelatin and other trace minerals. Marrow provides vitamin A, vitamin K2, minerals including zinc, iron, boron, manganese, and selenium, as well as Omega-3 and Omega-6 fatty acids. Include fresh vegetables. Use Apple Cider Vinegar to draw out extra valuable nutrients. Babies have fewer digestive problems when naturally derived gelatine and trace minerals are included in their diet.
8. **Limit certain foods upon becoming aware of their addictive qualities**, such as junk food cravings. Start by clearing away the cupboard of unhealthy options. Food can be donated; it doesn't have to be disposed.
9. **Don't skip meals.** Starving the body triggers deprivation, and your body will slow down its metabolism believing it is not receiving enough food.
10. **Stop and ask yourself if you are really hungry.** Question any desire to overeat.
11. **Drink plenty of water.**
12. **Read the food labels.** Always check the proper serving size.
13. **Change the way your food is prepared.** The use of fresh herbs like oregano, mint, thyme, and rosemary can enhance flavors. Eat more whole foods and fewer foods that are processed, refined, and packaged.

14. **Keep in mind that quick weight-loss diets are often costly, impractical, and many have unbalanced restrictions.** Make healthy adaptations to your current meals, and keep these changes as an ongoing lifestyle choice.
15. **Switch to oatmeal; eat more fresh vegetables and whole grain bread.**
16. **Remember that raw foods contain the most nutrients.** You may want to consider getting some seasonal vegetable plants from the nursery and growing those vegetables yourself. These plants do not require large spaces. They can be placed on window sills, balconies, kitchen tops, and left to grow in a pot. Growing and nurturing your own vegetables can inspire and motivate new habits that nourish your body.
17. **Treats are usually associated with a sweet reward. Reconsider this tendency.** Before obesity became a global issue and eating became recreation, people spent more time engaged in activities that were satisfying to both the body and their emotional selves. While we eat food to nourish our bodies, our emotions also need nourishment—a sense of belonging, feeling safe, love, and respect. Physical activity is a good way to promote the release of happy hormones that boost mental and emotional well-being.
18. **Watch for any food intolerances.** Symptoms can range from digestive problems, mood swings, tiredness, and bloating. Record the symptoms, what and when you ate, and what occurred. Consult your doctor if this is an ongoing issue.
19. **Depending on what mothers eat, babies in the womb can become accustomed to a variety of flavors.** The taste of the amniotic fluid changes according to your diet.
20. **Remember that you are working with your body to experience a wonderful pregnancy.** It may be a good idea to invest in your well-being by exploring your food options with a Nutritional Therapist.

21. **Try not to get frustrated.** Be patient and give yourself time to adjust.
22. **Review any medication with your healthcare provider.** This includes any prescriptions or over-the-counter medications, supplements, and herbs.

Avoid

1. **Processed food.** Nutrition is processed out.
2. **Commercially fried foods.** These have a high fat and calorie content. The composition of hydrogenated oil changes as it is reused, breaking down and causing more oil to be absorbed into food. Homemade fried foods are a better option as an occasional indulgence.
3. **Hydrogenated vegetable oils** such as margarine and industrially processed vegetable oils. Use of these oils has been linked to several adverse health conditions including impaired blood sugar control, inflammation and harm to heart health.
4. **Foods low in certain nutrients.** Your body may burn less calories and store fat.
5. **Artificial sweeteners, monosodium glutamate, and additives.** Many of these additives have been linked to a higher risk of metabolic syndrome and gastrointestinal distress.
6. **Cigarettes, alcohol, and drugs.** Smoking raises the risk of birth defects and congenital heart defects. Alcohol can pass from the mother's blood into the baby's blood. It can damage and harm the growth of the baby's cells. Drugs can create behavioral and cognitive problems in a child. The baby may be born dependent on the drug as well.

For any changes to occur, you have to let go of old habits. With a new life on the horizon, you are working on making a deeper connection with your body. Making small changes removes some of the pressure and feelings of being overwhelmed. It is easier to manage and adopt incremental change, and this accumulative process will grow into remarkable overall lifestyle shifts. Choose one small habit now, and adopt a new healthy choice without excuses.

Keep a Journal to Monitor the Food-Mood Connections

Emotions are common eating triggers. The need to belong, feel safe, and feel good about ourselves is as important as the food that physically sustains us. Food is often used to pacify feelings of worthlessness, frustration, anger, or unhappiness. Food can be used as a distraction, or to pass away time or deal with boredom. Empty, greasy, and sugary calories taste good, and such foods are easy to turn to for comfort.

- Do you eat when you are feeling lonely or cut off?
- Do you eat when you are angry?
- Do you eat when you are worried?
- Do you eat when you feel overwhelmed?
- Do you eat because the clock says it's meal time?

Keeping a journal for several days can help you see any common patterns.
Record any events that sparked your emotions which triggered unhealthy eating.
Record when, where, and what you ate.

Emotions influence our mood and behavior. We can address our eating habits, and find comfort in adopting new lifestyle choices, without turning to unhealthy food options.

Examples:

- After dealing with a difficult co-worker, or after an argument with a loved one, I felt the need to eat some chocolate to make myself feel good.
- I had thirty minutes to wait for an appointment, so I decided to have a milkshake to occupy my time.

Food Journal: Connecting Foods and Moods

Date: _____

You crave an unhealthy comfort food.
Why do you feel this urge to eat? Describe the situation or circumstances around the time of your food choice.

_____
_____
_____
_____.

Describe your mood.

_____
_____
_____
_____.

Are you eating because the clock says it's meal time?

_____
_____
_____
_____.

List what you eat, and how much.

_____
_____

_____
_____.

Were you hungry at the time, or just craved the food?
_____
_____
_____
_____.

Describe any challenges or emotions you felt. Can you find ways to address these stressors or feelings directly, without turning to food?
_____
_____
_____
_____.

    Breaking any habit will require you to make some effort. Whenever you see or feel a perceived self-limitation, reframe the sentiment into a question. Challenge the idea and see if it is relevant. Ask yourself, "How can I overcome this?" Take small steps, and follow through with each until you have formed a new habit.

20

The Benefits of Exercise

Yoga, Pilates, walking, regular swimming, or moderate exercises (within comfortable limits) are beneficial during pregnancy and the postpartum period. Good health is maintained by exercising four to five times per week, for at least thirty minutes each time. There are also specific exercises for pregnancy, including pelvic muscle exercises (also known as Kegel exercises), pelvic rocking, and squatting.

Regular exercise can help you to cope with the physical changes. As pregnancy progresses, the mother's center of gravity changes. The new distribution of weight on the abdomen can add strain to the back. I recommend joining a prenatal exercise class, or consulting a trainer who has expertise in developing programs for pregnant woman, to help with stretching and maternal centering. Please also consult with your health provider before you embark on any exercise program.

7 Benefits of Exercise

1. Reduces backaches, constipation, bloating, and swelling.
2. Promotes an easier, less-complicated labor and quicker recovery.
3. Improves cardiovascular function.
4. Boosts your mood and energy levels.

5. Helps you relax and sleep better.
6. Prevents excess weight gain.
7. Promotes muscle tone, strength, and endurance.

If you have not exercised for a while, start with shorter periods and build up to reach at least thirty minutes a day. If you are a beginner, walking, swimming, and other low-impact aerobics can be a great place to start. Remember to warm up, stretch, and cool down. Drink plenty of water to stay hydrated. You should be able to carry on a conversation while exercising. Not being able to speak is an indication that you are pushing yourself too hard.

Squatting—Learn to squat and build the muscles on your legs. Squatting opens the pelvis and can help move the baby into the ideal birthing position.

Avoid

Kickboxing—This can cause trauma to the abdomen.

Exercising at high altitudes—Symptoms of high-altitude illness include headaches, nausea, and fatigue. High altitude reduces the amount of oxygen in the blood, which also means your baby will receive less oxygen. This can cause you and your fetus to develop hypoxia, which can lead to developmental problems.

Scuba diving—This puts the baby at risk of decompression sickness.

Benefits of a Birthing Ball

A birthing ball can be used for the following:

- Strengthening and supporting the lower back.
- Sitting upright on the birthing ball can help to open up the pelvis and loosen the ligaments.
- Helping to relieve back pain.
- Staying balanced on the ball strengthens the pelvis muscles.
- Improving posture.
- Getting the baby into a better position during labor.

Ways to Stay Motivated

- Take short walks in your neighborhood.
- Choose an activity that you enjoy.
- Join a class that fits your schedule.

21

What to Consider before Preparing Your Birth Plan

Each labor and childbirth is unique. Even from one pregnancy to the next, your experience can be completely different. Understanding the outcomes you would like, as well as how you wish to interact with your healthcare provider, can help them to make decisions in line with your expectations.

A birth plan should be obtainable from your healthcare provider. An exercise is also included later in this chapter to help you create and refine your own birth plan. If you have any questions, or if you feel unsure and uncomfortable with any part of the plan, please discuss this with your healthcare provider or birthing caregiver, and obtain a second opinion. I encourage you to undertake an Active Birth. A birth plan should communicate *your* wishes, preferences, and goals.

Labor Pains Have a Purpose

Pain is a normal part of labor. Throughout your labor, pain is dynamic and changes as the experience progresses. As the contractions become closer and more intense, the pain becomes more purposeful and meaningful. You are moving closer towards embracing your baby!

Hormones are chemical messengers that originate in our brains, and they cascade signals to other parts of our bodies. These chemical messengers have a powerful influence on both our emotional and physical states. Labor and the process of childbirth involve peak levels of pregnancy and lactation hormone, *prolactin,* and a happy hormone, *oxytocin,* within the mother. *Beta-endorphins* are produced by our bodies as a natural painkiller. *Epinephrine* and *norepinephrine,* also known as adrenaline and noradrenaline, are fight or flight stress hormones that are released during labor. The release of all these hormones is vital to the whole labor process, and this is strongly linked to our primordial feelings of safety. Labor can stall or slow down when stress hormones are activated earlier by feelings of fear or uncertainty. It is important to emotionally prepare and practice for labor, as you have done in the previous exercises, as well as to have a birth plan that reaffirms your desires during labor.

Oxytocin signals the uterus to begin contracting during early-stage labor, while also signalling the brain to produce pain-reducing beta-endorphins. Oxytocin and endorphin levels are highest at the time of natural birth, and they play a large role in the feelings of euphoria and receptiveness of a mother to her newborn baby. Many mothers report feeling more connected to the experience of birth with this natural rush of hormones. Oxytocin is also responsible for the strong contractions that allow the separation of the placenta from the uterus. Strongest contractions occur when oxytocin levels are high, and this in turn reduces the likelihood of bleeding or post-partum hemorrhage.

The fight or flight *catecholamine* hormones, epinephrine and norepinephrine, play an important role in the second stage of labor as birth occurs. These hormones give a mother a burst of energy to allow her to strongly push. As the level of fight or flight hormones increase, the release of *prostaglandin* and *cortisol* are also stimulated to further contractions. Cortisol and the catecholamines largely prepare the baby for the transition to self-breathing. They are the primary mediator hormones that coordinate the clearance of fetal lung fluid and surfactant secretions. This process allows the baby to clear amniotic fluid from its lungs, and for consistent breathing to occur. Catecholamines trigger the breakdown of glycogen in the baby to produce energy, while also regulating the baby's heart and breathing rates, helping them to more effectively cope with the strong contractions of birthing.

Prolactin increases as pregnancy progresses and peaks at the start of labor. It is also produced during and after labor, preparing a mother for breastfeeding. When combined with oxytocin, it helps with the bonding between a mother and newborn baby.

Labor pains are normal and part of a typical birth. Pain should not be perceived as a physiological threat to you or your baby. Our bodies have well-adjusted feedback mechanisms to deal with pain, and they only require self-trust in their purpose. Pain is challenging. The unleashing of its intensity can make you feel powerless, and it can distract you from its overall function. I encourage you to learn and practice ways to trust your body, and to follow this natural internal process.

Pain is a marker for how your labor is progressing, and it is a trigger for hormones that continue to advance birthing. Rather than trying to control the process, reach into your inner capacity and follow the rhythm of your body. Understand, prepare, and practice for the process. You have the capacity to extend inwardly, and to find the strength needed to break through any limitations.

Labor and childbirth is not something you have to do by yourself. There is strength in unity and alignment of needs. Reassurance comes in the form of love and encouragement from your partner and/or family, as well as in choosing the right birthing caregiver. Knowing that you have someone you can trust beside you amplifies your ability to cope. It soothes any anxiety, boosts your confidence, and gives you the best chance of a natural birth with good outcomes.

There are several complementary techniques that may help you to manage pain (see "Pain Management" section starting on page 105), with less effect on the natural process. Develop a birth plan that includes a few alternatives, so that you have a plan for changing circumstances. Labor and childbirth should unfold spontaneously, while ensuring the safety and health of you and your baby. Your caregiver is there to support and encourage you. Your birth plan is there to ensure your preferences are known.

Hospitals & Birthing Centers

The management approach of hospitals and birthing centers determines the extent to which parents can make decisions, or choices, during the birth of their child. Take a tour of a hospital or birthing center before committing to using their services. Learn about their policies and procedures. Check whether the hospital or birthing center can accommodate your birth plan and preferences.

Styles of Management

Active management describes the approach your caregiver will follow to ensure the outcome of a birth. There is often a fixed timeframe, usually birth within twelve hours. If the expectant mother has not spontaneously gone into labor within her due date period, active management will favor induction. However, it is beneficial for you to labor naturally. You and the baby benefit from the natural hormones of labor.

Expectant management follows a "wait and watch" approach. The well-being of mother and baby is monitored, and intervention is only taken if and when a problem is identified.

Environment

A hospital or birthing center should have a calm, relaxed, and comfortable environment where a mother feels safe and supported. The type of environment has a large effect on hormone release, and the progression of labor. Oxytocin release, and its effectiveness, is greater when the neocortex is not being stimulated by bright lights, people speaking, or strong odors. Soft lighting and a quiet environment also stimulate the production of *melatonin,* making your body feel more restful.

Freedom of Movement

Mothers feel more comfortable during labor when they are able walk around and change positions as desired, without being confined by policies or restrictions of space. The term "Active Birth" refers to the way a mother is effectively involved during labor, moving into comfortable positions and making informed decisions as needed. You may decide that upright positions feel more comfortable and help you to better cope with the pain. This may involve walking, standing, swaying, or moving your hips. You can remain upright during labor to ensure that pressure on the perineum is being applied in the correct location. If your caregivers indicate that the baby is lying in a posterior position, you will be able to try some forward leaning positions that encourage the baby to turn.

Choose a place where you feel free to work with your body, and in positions that are best for you. Freedom of movement will allow you to practice different natural positions, in order to arrive at a good outcome.

Pain Management

Pain management techniques include *acupressure, visualisation, hypnosis, massage, yoga*, and *partner support*. You have become familiar with some of these practices through earlier exercises.

Your uterus is a collection of muscles, all performing at peak process during birth. Muscles function best when we are well hydrated, well nourished, and receive a good oxygen supply. Drink plenty of liquids, and remember to breathe deeply. It is important to choose a hospital or birthing center that will support your pain management preferences.

Touch—This could be Reiki, massage, or simply having someone to hold your hand.

A massage works by reducing tension in an area. A firm massage using the palms to apply pressure on the lower back is an effective reliever of back pain. Long, firm strokes along the outer thighs are helpful during transition (the last stage of labor), especially if the mother's legs are shaking. Firm hip pressure via massage, towards the end of labor, can relieve tension felt in the pelvis.

Water immersion—A warm bath or having a shower can be very soothing. A shower should be prepared with a fitting chair or stool in advance. Ensure that the surface is non-slip. Sit on the chair or stool in the shower, and direct the flow of water to your abdomen or back. A bath tub should preferably be deep enough to immerse your abdomen. Most hospitals and birthing centers are equipped with these facilities, and your caregiver should be present to assist you.

Hot packs—These help your body release natural painkiller endorphins.

Birthing ball—Use a birthing ball to reduce the weight on your legs, and to relax your back. The ball can be used to help you stretch, reach more comfortable positions, or practice movements to rotate the baby into an anterior position. The anterior position is where the baby's head is down in the pelvis, facing the mother's back, and is the best position for labor.

Rebozo—A Rebozo is a traditional cloth used for comfort during pregnancy in Mexico and Latin America. Gentle use of a Rebozo promotes movement, relaxation and physical support during later pregnancy. During labor, the Rebozo cloth is tenderly moved from side to side to provide a pleasant rhythmic movement of the pelvis. This sifting movement, known as "manteada" (meaning "body rocking"), may facilitate some useful movement of the baby during labor.

The Rebozo technique may also be used to re-position a breech baby for birth. "Acomodada" (meaning "to accommodate"), is the process of wrapping a laboring mother in a Rebozo cloth to help attain the best position of a baby for birth.

You should always talk to your healthcare provider about whether it's safe for you to use a Rebozo, and which techniques will provide the greatest support based on your particular circumstances.

Delivery

Natural or Vaginal Birth (also referred to as Unmedicated Vaginal Delivery)

The first stage of labor begins when you feel regular contractions. These contractions cause the cervix to dilate and soften, while also making it shorter and thinner. The first stage of labor is the longest of the three stages. Early labor is unpredictable, and you may want to stay at home and work with your partner or caregiver to manage the pain until your contractions increase in frequency and intensity. Laboring in a more tranquil setting, away from the frequent monitoring of hospital or birthing center staff, is much more comfortable. Use self-hypnosis, affirmations, meditation, music, and other techniques to relax.

Remember to move around to encourage your labor to progress. Standing, walking, squatting, sitting, and swaying ease tension and allow the weight of the baby to press on the cervix. This encourages the cervix to open. Avoid lying on your back where possible, as this places pressure on major arteries. It is okay to lie down. Use a pillow to form a wedge so that you are lying slightly to one side if you want to sleep. Keep your lower leg straight, bend your upper knee, and rest it on a pillow. This position opens up the pelvis and encourages the baby to rotate and descend. You can also use a hot compress, massage, or acupressure to make yourself feel more comfortable.

Keep yourself well hydrated and nourished. The length of early labor can vary from hours to days. You are working with your body to birth your baby. The freedom to follow your body's rhythm and move can make labor easier and faster. If your water breaks, or if you experience vaginal bleeding, call your healthcare provider immediately. During early labor, the cervix softens, thins, and eventually dilates. Active labor begins when the cervix is dilated to about six centimeters (roughly the width of three fingers). Your healthcare provider or caregiver should be present by this stage.

Elective Labor Induction

Elective labor induction is the initiation of labor within a set date. During the latter part of pregnancy, the presenting part of the baby applies pressure to the mother's cervix. This pressure, when evenly applied to the cervix, triggers the mother's brain to release increased levels of oxytocin which stimulates contractions. If labor is induced, your body and baby may not be ready to produce natural oxytocin to begin contractions. The drug *Pitocin* may be recommended to you in order progress labor. Pitocin has the potential to create intense and frequent contractions, and reduce the oxygen supply to the baby. Doctors may recommend a C-section if the baby becomes distressed.

Full-term pregnancy is considered between thirty-nine weeks, and forty weeks and six days. Trust your body's timing, but do check with your medical professional and caregiver if you do not go into natural labor in this timeframe. Your healthcare provider should evaluate several factors concerning your health, and the baby's health, before determining if any induction is necessary. A labor induction may be recommended by your healthcare provider if there are concerns about your health or the baby's health.

Caesarean Delivery or C-Section

This is a surgical procedure used to deliver a baby through an incision made in the abdomen and uterus. The procedure will be planned ahead if you have had a previous C-section, or if you have developed any complications.

A C-Section may be recommended by your healthcare provider when:

1. A baby (or babies) is in an abnormal position.
2. A baby is distressed.
3. You are carrying twins, and the lead baby is in an abnormal position.
4. There are health concerns—a prolapsed umbilical cord, a problem with the placenta, or fibroids obstructing the birth canal.

A C-Section is discouraged if you plan to have other children. The procedure increases the risk of breathing problems in a newborn, along with an increased risk of infections, blood clots, reaction to anaesthesia, and post-partum hemorrhaging in the mother.

Pain Relief

Nitrous Oxide is a pain-relief drug that has no known effects on the natural, physiological progression of labor. It is considered relatively safe to use in low concentrations during labor. When you inhale nitrous oxide, only a small fraction is metabolized by the body, and the majority is released as you exhale. Nitrous oxide works by decreasing the sensation of pain, and it stimulates the release of natural hormones which reduce stress and anxiety. It does not interfere with your body's ability to release oxytocin. Nitrous oxide has not been seen to cross the placenta, or interfere with the baby's alertness, breastfeeding or bonding with a mother immediately after birth. Some women may feel dizzy or nauseous for short periods while they inhale the gas. These brief side effects usually discontinue within a few minutes after they stop.

Sterile Water Injections (SWI) —Sterile water papules are small injections of water, administered just beneath the skin on your lower back. SWI has no effect on the baby or your mobility, and it is an effective method for relieving back pain during labor.

Epidural—Local anaesthetics are injected via a catheter into a small space outside the spinal cord on the lower back. Epidurals manage the pain of childbirth by blocking out the nerve signals for pain in your lower spine. The size of your pelvis, baby's size and position can impact on the level of pain. During an unmedicated birth, oxytocin levels gradually increase and are highest around the time of birth. This peak level is largely triggered by the sensations of stretching and contraction of the birth canal as the baby is born. The same high peak level of oxytocin often does not occur when an epidural is in place, interfering with the normal cascade of birth hormones.

1. If you decide on an epidural, a catheter is inserted once the epidural is administered. After you have an epidural, sensations in your lower body are minimized, and you are unable to change positions when it may be beneficial to do so. If you cannot feel your contractions, you cannot push at the right time and with enough force to help the baby move.
2. An epidural can slow down labor. Pitocin is administered to push labor along and strengthen contractions. Epidurals can cause a sudden drop in blood pressure in the mother. This may result in less oxygen-rich blood being pumped to baby. It also increases the overall risk of birth where forceps or vacuum assistance is required.
3. Continuous electronic monitoring, a local anaesthetic, and an intravenous line confine you to bed.
4. Research indicates that perineal tears are more common when an epidural is used.
5. Babies can develop respiratory depression following an epidural.
6. An epidural can interfere with the normal cascade of birth hormones.

The cascade of interventions—When birth begins and continues spontaneously in its own time, you are less likely to require interventions. Any unnecessary intervention has the potential to lead to more interventions, and further complications.

Episiotomy—This is a surgical procedure of cutting the perineum to provide more space for the baby to be born. Epidurals have been seen to increase the risk of episiotomies. Numerous studies recommend that episiotomies should only be restrictively used.

Medication during childbirth—Pain relief medication can cause babies to be less alert, and less able to orient themselves. A newborn baby liver will work to process any drugs that have been introduced into their system. Additional side effects may include central nervous system depression, respiratory depression, and a decrease in ability to regulate body temperature. Pain relievers, or anesthesia, have also been seen to contribute to breastfeeding problems. The baby and mother may be drowsy, and delay the first nursing.

Cord clamping—Delayed clamping can be greatly beneficial to newborns, especially premature babies. Clamping is usually delayed to between one and five minutes after birth. This delay lets blood continue to flow from the placenta to the newborn after delivery, and it is usually sufficient time for blood to circulate to the baby.

The placenta—In some culture, the placenta is kept for its healing and spiritual benefits. There are beautiful ceremonies held to thank, and celebrate, this "Tree of Life" before it is buried. A tree is often planted at a later date to commemorate the ritual. Eating the placenta is still practiced in some parts of the world, and in Chinese medicine, it is considered to have medicinal value. The placenta can also be dehydrated and encapsulated. If you are unsure what to do with your placenta, you may ask for it to be kept until you decide.

Newborn Care

Skin to skin contact—A baby that is held skin-to-skin on a mother's chest has better temperature control, and often better blood sugar regulation. Studies have found that breastfeeding is more successful when mothers are permitted to stay skin-to-skin with their newborn babies for longer initial periods. Babies who are breastfed within the first thirty minutes to an hour of being born find it much easier to learn how to latch. Babies have an innate nature to suckle and feed. Once a baby is placed skin-to-skin, between its mother's bare breasts after delivery, it will find the breast, latch, and start nursing.

Bathing baby—Benefits of delaying a newborn's first bath:

1. **Reduces the risk of infection:** *Vernix* is a white, creamy protective coating on a baby's skin that stabilizes temperature, and acts as an antimicrobial and moisturizer. You may want to delay the bath and allow sufficient time for baby's skin to absorb the vernix.
2. **Stabilizes infant blood sugar:** In the first few hours after birth, a baby has to adjust to life outside the uterus. Your baby loses it source of blood sugar from the placenta. Bathing a baby too soon after birth can cause low blood sugar. If bathing causes crying and stress, this releases stress hormones which cause a baby's blood sugar to drop. This can make a baby too sleepy to wake up and breastfeed.
3. **Temperature control:** Giving a baby a bath too soon can cause hypothermia. The temperature inside the womb was approximately 98.6° F, or 37° C. A baby uses a significant amount of energy to keep warm in the first few hours after birth. If the baby gets cold, its blood sugar can drop or it can experience other complications. Delayed bathing is not a protocol in all hospitals, but you can request it.
4. **Bathing products:** Inquire about the bathing products used at the hospital or birthing center in advance. Arrange to purchase your own product if you prefer. You may also ask to be involved with the first bath.

Rooming in—When "rooming in," the baby's crib is kept at the side of a mother's bed in the post-labor recovery room. This helps the breastfeeding mother to understand cues for when a baby is hungry or sleepy. The process is helpful to learn baby behaviors for when you leave the hospital or birthing center.

Diapers for baby—Inquire if the hospital or birthing center will provide baby diapers for the duration of stay, or if you need to purchase and provide your own.

22

Create Your Birth Plan

A *birth plan* is a simple tool used to communicate your preferences to your medical professional and caregivers. Use the information detailed in "What to Consider Before Preparing Your Birth Plan" to create a plan that details what you would like to happen before, during, and after labor. A care team has limited time. A clear one-page plan is the most effective way to identify and communicate your preferences to the team.

Hospitals and birthing centers have their own policies. It might be helpful to establish and understand your caregiver's approach earlier to know if they conflict with your ideas. A birth plan is a helpful tool to explore your options.

While birth is a normal biological process, and medical intervention can save lives, you may want to explore all your options—especially for during labor. This is an opportunity to become informed, understand, and choose any options available to you, instead of simply consenting at the time.

Birth Plan

Name:_____

Due Date:_____

Practitioner's Name:_____

Support Persons:_____

Health Factors: Identify any health issues, allergies, or concerns:
_____
_____
_____
_____.

My planned delivery preferences

(Please refer to the notes below and the chapter "What to Consider before Preparing Your Birth Plan".)

1._____
_____
_____
_____.

2._____
_____
_____
_____.

3._____
_____
_____
_____.

4._____
_____
_____
_____.

5._____
_____
_____
_____.

6._____
_____
_____
_____.

7._____
_____
_____
_____.

8._____
_____
_____
_____.

9._____
_____
_____
_____.

1. Focus on the outcomes and strategies you would prefer to use once you are in labor.
2. Detail your preferences for pain management and pain relief. What techniques would you like to use to help yourself cope

with labor pains? References to any specific techniques, and prior practice with your support person, will make these techniques easier to follow.
3. Describe the role of your partner, support person, or family members during labor.
4. Describe anything you would like to repeat or avoid from previous births.
5. Carefully consider your decisions on the use of medication. Informed consent for the use of medication means you are aware of the name and reason for the drug, and its potential risk and benefits. Make time to ask questions during your prenatal exams.
6. Proposed Labor Interventions:
   Are you aware of the reason for any possible procedure or other intervention, and its potential risk and benefits? If not, find out.
   What would happen if you do not agree with the proposed intervention? What would happen if you waited?
   What alternative(s) exist to the proposed therapy?
   It is appropriate to ask questions unless there is an emergency. Ask for time to make your decision.
7. Cord clamping—Be specific about timing. For example, the cord is to remain unclamped until the placenta is born.
8. What would you like to do with the placenta?
9. Describe your preferences for newborn care.

23

Postpartum Essential List

This is a list of suggested essentials that you may want to arrange during your pregnancy.

1. **Peri bottle**—After delivery your entire perineum is swollen and sore. This squirt bottle allows you to clean this sensitive area. You are able control water pressure and direction with ease. This is especially comforting if you have had stitches.

2. **Maternal pad for Lochia**—*Lochia* is a combination of blood, placenta tissue, bacteria, cells, and mucus released by the wound where the placenta tears away from the uterine wall. This natural process takes about six to eight weeks as the womb returns to its normal size. It is part of your postpartum healing. Breastfeeding and massaging the uterus speed up the process. It is a good idea to stock up on comfortable maxi pads.

3. **Padsicles**—A *padsicle* is a pad prepared and stored in your freezer. This pad is then placed inside your underwear to relieve pain. You will need witch hazel without alcohol, 100% pure lavender oil, and 100% pure unscented Aloe Vera gel. To make a padsicle, lay enough tin foil to wrap each pad on a clean counter. Place the pad on foil and spread the Aloe Vera using the back of a clean spoon

across the pad. Add one or two drops of lavender oil. Spray or gently pour witch hazel over the pad. Do not over-saturate. Wrap up the pads individually, place them in a storage container or bag, and store in the freezer. To manage a heavy flow, thick sanitary napkins are best.

4. **Prepared homemade meals**—Prepare a good balance of nutrient-dense freezer meals. Heading for the kitchen straight after childbirth to make a meal is the last thing you want to do. Store the food in glassware for easy heating in the oven. According to the FDA, cooked meat, such as lamb, pork, and beef, should not be kept frozen for longer than two months. Cooked chicken can be frozen up to four months.

5. **Weighted blanket**—Sleeping under a weighted blanket has a calming effect. It can help soothe your over-stimulated nerves so that you can sleep. Consult the weight chart to find the right size blanket for your body.

6. **Belly support**—A belly binder or wrap encourages your body to return to its shape. Check with your doctor if this is suitable for you.

7. **Wash the baby's clothes**—A newborn baby's clothes should be washed before use. Clothes are stored in warehouse that may also house bugs. Clothes can be treated with formaldehyde to keep them looking fresh during shipping. Blankets and swaddle blankets should also be washed.

8. **Nursing pads**—This is for breastfeeding moms. Nursing pads are handy for drips.

9. **Baby bottles**—Use a smaller bottle with a stage 1 slow-flow nipple to control how fast milk is released. As the baby grows and the quantity increases, a bigger bottle with a stage 2 nipple for a faster flow is better.

10. **Baby monitors**—These are helpful for keeping an eye on the baby while you are busy.

11. **Nursing pillow**—The pillow eases the strain on your back and arms and comforts the baby during feed time. Some are C-shaped or U-shaped to snuggle against your stomach, and some wrap all the way around your waist. Choose a style that suits you. Some pillows have an adjustable strap or belt that allow a customized fit. Removable pillowcases will make cleaning your pillow much easier.

12. **Breast pumps**—Some birthing centers or hospitals now encourage mothers to bring breast pumps. On-staff lactation consultants can assist and answer any questions.

13. **A postpartum sealing ceremony**—This is a powerful nurturing ceremony that leaves you feeling nurtured, safe, and cared for. It begins with a bath that is a modification of traditional Mexican *Temazcal,* or what is known as a "Sweat Lodge." The sealing ceremony is a tremendous way to support a mother as she reflects on the birth experience, and releases any tension from the body or trauma experienced. It is a time to simply relax and allow oneself to be pampered. The ceremony begins as mother bathes in a water tub with freshly harvested herbs. The final sealing process involves *Rebozo* or a "bone closing" ceremony. Herbal oils are used to gently massage the body, starting at the feet and ending at the head. The final touch is a womb massage and belly binding with abdominal bandages. This should be done late in the

evening so that the mother can go straight to bed. The Sealing Ceremony realigns the mother physically and energetically.

14. **A postpartum bath mix**—Make with comfrey, uva-ursi, and Himalayan Pink salts. The mix makes aches and pains melt away. To prepare: Place 1/3 cup of the herbs in boiling water and allow them to steep for twenty minutes. Strain and add the resulting liquid to bath water, along with a tablespoon of Himalayan pink salt. Ensure that your products are obtained from a reputable supplier. If you have any allergies, a warm shallow bath of only water is just as comforting.

24

The Three Stages of Labor

Your body has been tirelessly at work preparing for labor. The middle range for labor is between twelve and eighteen hours for your first child, and slightly shorter for subsequent babies. The first phase is the longest, and labor begins with *early labor* (Stage One), followed by *active labor* (Stage Two), and *transition* (Stage Three). Labor starts quietly, builds progressively with early contractions, and ends with a complete dilation of the cervix. Few labors begin with spontaneous water breaking.

If you think that you are going into labor, avoid spending time by yourself. Call to inform your family, friends, partner or healthcare provider.

Stage One—Early Labor

During early labor, you may experience backache, lower abdominal pressure, indigestion, diarrhea, blood-tinged mucous discharge, or your water may break (although this is usually during active labor). In early labor, contractions become regular, and they do not go away with a change of position or activity. Try a short brisk walk, and then lie down to rest. You may experience moderate contractions that last for about thirty-five to forty seconds. If the contractions are consistent during walking and resting, then it is very likely that your labor has begun. Alert your partner and your doctor.

Contractions will progressively build to become longer in duration, lasting sixty seconds. They will grow stronger in sensation and closer together. Contractions occur every four to eight minutes in early labor.

With the onset of contractions, your cervix begins the process of *effacing* (becoming thin and soft) and *dilating* (opening wide for the baby to pass through). The cervix must efface considerably before it starts dilating. Effacement is estimated in percentage. Dilation is estimated in centimeters.

As your baby descends into the pelvis, the pressure from their head on your cervix will aid in dilation. You should be at the birthing center, or your midwife should already be present as your cervix dilates to six centimeters. The baby is fully engaged when their head is low and pressing on your cervix.

Stage Two—Active Labor

Your contractions will become longer, stronger, and closer together. Active labor starts when your contractions are regular and your cervix has six centimeters of dilation. This phase is short in comparison to early labor. Use your coping strategies and techniques to manage and work through each phase. As the contractions become intense, you will find it difficult to distract yourself from their sensations, as the time of rest between each shortens. Contractions last for forty seconds to sixty seconds, becoming more frequent and occurring every three to four minutes.

You will feel increasing pain and discomfort with the contractions, including increasing backache, leg discomfort or heaviness, fatigue, increasing blood flow, and rupture of the membranes (commonly described as "water breaking."). Your confidence may waiver and you may find it difficult to relax. This is normal. Your partner or support person should be calm and strong, helping to assure you that you are going to make it through the process. Your partner or support person should always encourage you to try to keep going, even if they may have a hard time anticipating your needs. Ask for a massage, face towel, or whatever it is you may require. Stay hydrated.

Your body has now established a rhythm of contraction and dilation. Active labor may continue for thirty minutes to a couple of hours, before the transition begins. As labor progresses safely, your healthcare provider will only monitor you and allow you to work through your labor with your partner or support person.

Some babies require extra help to get into an optimal position to keep labor progressing steadily. Unless you are required to be in a specific position to allow close monitoring, continue changing positions or moving around to encourage your baby's descent. Do whatever relaxes you and makes you comfortable. Standing, squatting, kneeling, or being on all fours, are great positions to enhance the space available within the pelvis to encourage the baby's descent. The more your baby's head descends, the closer you are to achieving your goal of meeting your baby.

Stage Three—Transition

This is the final and most intense phase, where your cervix will be close to full dilation. If you are thinking of not using pain medication, your caregiver or support person should be able to offer some strategies on how to cope. Your caregiver may encourage you to take a shower or bath.

Transition can last between fifteen minutes and three hours. Contractions will be at the peak of intensity, lasting between sixty to ninety seconds long, and two to three minutes apart. Your body will exert extra effort pushing, and you may feel some pressure on your rectum. Being on all fours is a better position during this time. There is a surge of epinephrine (adrenaline). The effects of an epinephrine rush can include shaking, nausea, and sweating. With these sensations surging through your body, you may feel out of control or helpless. Once your cervix is fully dilated, your baby can pass through the pelvis, and twist its way out of the birth canal into the world! This phase is significantly shorter than the others.

Pushing and Delivery the Baby

There is a tremendous urge to push, and the contractions are intense. Push when instructed by your healthcare provider. Push as if you are experiencing a tremendous bowel movement, and rest between contractions. When the baby's head begins to crown, your healthcare provider may ask you to slow down your pushing to allow your baby's head and shoulders to emerge gently.

Congratulations! Rest and bond with your baby!

Delivery of the Placenta

Once the baby is born, the hard work is over! Your baby may be placed on your chest for immediate skin-to-skin contact. Your healthcare provider will attend to you and your baby according to the details on your birth plan. The umbilical cord is cut. You will feel some contraction again between five minutes and thirty minutes, when your body is ready to deliver the placenta. A few gentle pushes are required. This is the final stage that you have spent months preparing for!

25

Postpartum

Postpartum refers to the first six weeks after childbirth. You may be feeling less tolerant from the exhaustion of labor, and unsure about what you are doing. I want to assure you that you are not alone in your experience! Be patient with yourself, your baby and other loved ones. Early parenthood can feel overwhelming. Your body is adjusting, healing, and you are tired. You will spend much of your time feeding and comforting your baby. If this is your first child, you will soon learn to understand and respond to a baby's cues. You will eventually fall into a routine. Please continue with your meditation and affirmations. The continued practice will help you settle and transition into your new phase of motherhood.

Connect to Your Source of Inner Strength Daily

Find a quiet space. Make yourself comfortable and close your eyes. Take three full breaths into your abdomen. Visualize that every inhalation is calming. With every exhalation, release any tension, discomfort, and anxiety that you may feel. Take a few moments to relax. Set your intentions for the day—feel love in your heart, strength in your body, and joy with your baby.

Postpartum Care

Vaginal soreness—To ease discomfort:

- Cool the area by using an ice pack or padsicle (described earlier in the Postpartum Essential List).
- Use a squeeze bottle to pour warm water over the area as you pass urine.
- Sit in a warm bath that is deep enough to cover your hips and buttocks.

Vaginal discharge—This discharge is made up of blood and the superficial mucous membrane that lined your uterus during pregnancy. It will be red and heavy in the beginning, but will change to become watery pinkish-brown, and finally yellowish-white.

Contractions—Also referred to as "afterpains," these are common during breastfeeding. Your uterus is shrinking and the pain will subside with time.

Pain during bowel movements—Place a padsicle (containing witch hazel) on the area to provide some comfort between movements.

Sore muscles—This is common after labor. Rest as much as you can!

Breast engorgement—This may cause discomfort and swelling. Place a warm or cold compress, to relieve discomfort.

If you had a C-Section:

- Avoid strenuous activity.
- Avoid lifting anything heavier than your baby.
- Shower as usual and pat the incision dry.

Rest—The body must rest to heal. Stay warm and eat nutritious warm food. Include bone broths, meaty soups, or stews in your diet. Drink water and incorporate fruit, vegetables, and whole grains into your meal plans.

Acupuncture—According to ancient Chinese teachings, vital life energy circulates through the body along the meridians. The components of *qi* (energy), Yin energy and Yang energy, are constantly transforming. The ideal state of health is achieved naturally by balancing Yin and Yang in the body. Acupuncture can improve your general well-being and energy levels. It reduces pain, improves circulation, balances hormones, and relaxes you.

Grounding — The simple pleasure of walking barefoot, or lying on the ground and reconnecting with the Earth, has remarkable physiological benefits. Walking barefoot outside or sitting on the ground connects us to the Earth's conductive system, and transfers its electrons from the ground into our bodies. The Earth is electron-rich and your body benefits from this natural healing energy. The process reduces inflammation, speeds healing, and reduces pain. You feel connected and refreshed. Simply being outdoors can change your motivation and bring you fresh ideas.

Herbal remedies—I recommend consulting a holistic Naturopath during your pregnancy to discuss remedies that support your postpartum healing. *Prepare the suggested ingredients during your pregnancy, and have them ready for use postpartum.*

26

Breastfeeding

Your diet directly influences the composition of your milk during breastfeeding. It is not uncommon for woman to feel nutritionally depleted and drained after birth. A breastfeeding mother needs an additional 300 to 500 kilocalories (kcal) per day. Recent studies have shown that almond milk, fenugreek, ginger, and turmeric can increase the supply of breast milk without adverse effects. According to an article by Akkarach Bumrungpert et al in the journal *Breastfeeding Medicine*, a daily consumption of these ingredients after giving birth can increase the supply of nutritious breast milk by an enormous 100%.

Mama's Milk Tonic

This recipe includes ingredients that can increase a mother's milk supply after the delivery of her baby. The quantities below will produce two servings of the tonic.

Ingredients

- ¼ cup Almonds or almond meal (ground-up almond powder).
- 3 cups of warm water

- 1 teaspoon of ginger powder
- ½ teaspoon of fenugreek powder
- ½ teaspoon of cardamom powder
- ⅛ teaspoon of turmeric powder
- 2 dates (pitted)
- 1 tablespoon pure maple syrup

Directions

1. Add all ingredients to a blender, and blend on high for one minute or until well combined.
2. Make the recipe fresh daily, and drink warm for the first forty days after birth.

Nutrient-Dense Foods

A diet of nutrient-dense foods will provide essential sustenance in your breast milk for your growing baby. Eat suitable portions of foods such as eggs, liver, wild-caught salmon, leafy greens, berries, oats, quinoa, millet, beef, lamb, chicken, fish and roots vegetables. Fermented products like yogurt and kefir have beneficial probiotic effects. Raw fruit, vegetables and Camu camu powder are rich sources of vitamins, which can act as powerful antioxidants that strengthen your immune system.

Avoid

Avoid processed sugar, hydrogenated oils, soft drinks, junk food, cigarettes, drugs, and alcohol. Please check with healthcare provider that all of your prescription medication is safe for you to use while breastfeeding.

Certain Foods Can Decrease Milk Supply

Some foods have been seen to decrease breast milk supply. These include lemon balm, oregano, peppermint, sage, sorrel, black walnut, parsley, spearmint, thyme, and yarrow. Try to limit their quantities during breastfeeding.

Lactation Consultant

While breastfeeding has many health benefits for you and your baby, formula does save lives. Within eight hours of birth, your baby should be latching well and feeding every two hours. The associated pain and discomfort can make breastfeeding challenging. If you find yourself having trouble nursing, don't give up; see a lactation consultant where possible. A lactation consultant can teach you how to continue nursing comfortably.

The consultation usually includes a one-on-one assessment, and hands-on breastfeeding instruction. There is an examination of baby's oral anatomy, as well of your breasts and nipples. The consultant will watch your baby feed to observe the latch, and offer positioning assistance. You will be able to practice latching on your baby during the session, and learn how to tell when the baby is properly latched, drinking, and swallowing. Your partner may video the session on your phone so that you can become more familiar by replaying it.

Most consultants will weigh your baby before and after feeding using a very sensitive scale. This will help to determine how much breast milk is being ingested by the baby during feeding. You may ask any questions that you have, and address any specific breastfeeding concerns, during the consultation.

27

Bathing Baby

Bathing your baby is a wonderful way for any parent to bond with their newborn. The process may seem intimidating at first, but with a little preparation and practice, all parents are able to treasure and enjoy the experience. You are able to bath your baby at any time of the day. I recommend choosing a time when you are relaxed and won't be interrupted. If bathing relaxes your baby, you can use the experience and routine as a way to settle your baby for sleep. It is best to avoid bathing baby straight after feeding, or when baby is hungry.

Benefits

1. **Boosts the parent-baby bonding**—Bathing becomes a special moment of the day when you spend time together. Feeling your gentle touch lets the baby know that you care. Simply gazing into baby's eyes, and singing or talking sweetly, will let baby sense how much they are loved.
2. **Soothes a cranky baby**—The sensation of soaking in a warm bath is very calming and comforting.
3. **Induces sleep**—The feeling of being warm, loved and safe, puts baby in the mood to sleep.

Preparation for Bath Time

1. **Warm up the bathing room**—Babies lose body heat very quickly, especially when they are naked. The room should be warm, at least 80° F or 26° C before you start.
2. **Remove jewellery** and turn off your phone for a distraction-free bath.
3. **Gather essentials**—Gentle soap and shampoo, wash cloth, cotton balls, a clean plush towel, clean diaper, clean clothes, ointments and creams for after the bath, and a blanket. You want avoid walking around with a naked baby trying to gather items after a bath. Leave a towel open on a flat surface nearby so that it can be ready for use immediately after the bath.
4. **Water**—The water temperature should be warm and comfortable, around 100° F or 38° C. Use your elbow, or the inside of your wrist, to the test water temperature. These areas are more sensitive and accurate than your fingertips. Fill sufficient water in the tub to cover the bottom of the baby's body. *Never place the baby into the water while the faucet is still running. Never leave a baby unattended in the baby tub, and always keep one hand on your baby.*

Giving Baby a Bath

1. **A secure hold** will help your baby feel safe in the tub. Use your nondominant arm to support your baby's head and neck, and the other arm to hold and guide your baby's body into the water, feet first. Continue supporting your baby's head and back. You might also reach behind your baby and hold onto their opposite arm throughout the bath.

2. **Wash gently**—Hold baby securely under body, supporting their head and neck as before using one arm. Use mild soap sparingly, or no soap if you prefer, on most of the body. Do apply a little mild soap or cleanser to the diaper area if you are not using soap on the rest of baby's skin. Cotton balls are a great way to gently clean sensitive areas such as around the eyes. Dip a cotton ball into the water, and wipe one eye from the inner corner outward. Use another cotton ball, and do the same for the other eye. Use a wet cloth to wipe baby's face around the mouth, under the chin where milk can pool, inside and behind the ears. Continue washing under the neck, torso, and then underarms and between fingers. Make sure to wipe all creases and skin folds. Gently wipe across the head with a wash cloth. Wash the genitals. For girls, wipe with the wash cloth from front to back. For boys, simply wipe the area gently.
3. **Pat baby dry**—Gently pat baby dry. Thoroughly dry the bottom and any area where there are folds and creases. Avoid using powders as they can be an irritant. If you intend to apply baby lotion, place some in your palms and warm up the lotion before applying it. Dress the baby in clean clothes and diapers, and swaddle the baby in a blanket.
4. **Benefits of swaddling the baby**—Babies have a Moro reflex, also known as the startle reflex. Keeping your baby's arms bound in a swaddle can prevent this reflex from waking them up. Swaddling also reminds the baby of being in the comforts of the womb. Swaddling your baby is good for about six weeks.

Swaddling is definitely not recommended for babies once they can roll over.

Sponge Bath

If your baby's umbilical cord stump is still intact, or if a circumcised penis has not healed, give the baby a sponge bath. Place a soft towel or cloth on a bed or a counter, and use warm water, gentle soap, and a soft wash cloth to clean the baby's skin. Avoid open or unhealed skin areas. If the areas do get wet, dry them gently with a soft cloth. If a crust has formed around the stump, wipe it gently with sterile water and a clean soft cloth. The umbilical cord may take from three days, up to two weeks, to fall off.

28

Diapers

Diapers play a critical role in baby well-being. Newborns generally need to have their diapers changed ten to twelve times per day! Consistent diaper changes help to minimize diaper rash, infections or other hygiene related health problems. As with many aspects of parenthood, we are faced with a choice: cloth or disposable diapers. There are many aspects to consider (cost, ease of use, chemicals in products, environmental impact), but ultimately, your choice should be what is best for your baby and your particular household situation.

Disposable diapers have been a useful quick changing aid to many households, making life easier for parents. But disposable diapers are more costly in the long run, bad for the environment, and their use can sometimes irritate baby's skin. Modern cloth diapers have evolved and become far more efficient. They are no longer the sheets of cloth and safety clamps of the past. Their new stylish designs are sophisticated and easier to learn how to use.

Cloth diapers are comfortable to wear, easy to launder, and have no additional chemicals or fragrances.

Understanding Your Cloth Diaper

Modern reusable cloth diapers often have an inner absorbent layer, and an outer waterproof shell that looks and functions in a similar way to a disposable diaper.

The Absorbent layer—This part of the cloth diaper is highly absorbent and soaks up any wetness. It is made from a range of different fibers or fabrics such as bamboo, cotton microfiber, and hemp.

The Cover or Wrap—This part of the cloth diaper forms the outer shell and is waterproof. They are often made from PUL (polyurethane laminate), waterproofed nylon, vinyl, fleece or wool. Covers may have Velcro, snap closures, or be pull-over for easy fitting.

Inside the Diaper

Liner—A liner sits between the baby's skin and the absorbent layer. Liners are designed to hold solids, and form a barrier to the inner absorbent fibers. Rash creams and other ointments are often oily or thick in nature. These can clog the absorbent layer, making it less efficient. A liner will help to prevent solids or thick emulsions from entering the absorbent layer, making the diaper more effective and much easier to clean. Reusable liners can be washed, while disposable biodegradable liners can be thrown away or composted after flushing away solids.

Booster—Boosters can be added to further increase absorbency. These are made from multiple layers of fabric. They are great for heavy wetters and night-time use. A booster is usually inserted between the liner and the absorbent layer.

Newborn Styles

1. Fitted Diapers

A *Fitted Diaper* is made up of several absorbent layers that wrap around the baby's bottom, and it is fastened at the front with a snap-close fastener. This diaper requires a separate waterproof cover.

2. Flats and Prefolds

Flats are the traditional style of diaper. They are folded and fastened with a snap-close fastener.

Prefolds are a folded diaper with an extra absorbent layer stitched down the center of the diaper.

Flats and Prefold both require a waterproof cover.

Covers and Wraps— *These waterproof covers are used with fitted, flat, and prefold diapers.*

a. A *PUL* (polyurethane laminated) *cover* is a polyester fabric laminated to make the cover waterproof.
b. *Wool and fleece covers* are breathable, absorb moisture, and prevent leaks. Wool is usually the most expensive option, but is a natural material. It offers good breathability for increased air circulation (less irritation and rashes) and is anti-bacterial.

3. All-in-Ones (AIO)

These diapers incorporate an absorbent inner layer and an outer waterproofing in one product. These diapers have an adjustable closure at the waist, and are closest in style to disposable diapers.

How Many Diapers Would Your Baby Need?

Newborns may use between ten to twelve diapers per day.

While disposable diapers are a great part-time convenience, they make approximately 3.4 million tons of US landfill waste annually. Decomposing diapers produce methane and other toxic gases.

Diaper Rash

The causes can range from sensitive skin, fragrances (including in laundry detergent or cosmetics), and sensitivity to certain foods. Diapers should be changed regularly to prevent skin irritation.

The Best Treatment is Prevention

Time Out—Consider going without diapers whenever possible while the baby is awake. Wash your hands before diaper changes. Check diapers often, and change them immediately if wet or soiled. Use plain water to gently pat the area clean at every diaper change. A diaper lotion or cream can be applied using a cotton pad or cloth to gently cleanse baby's bottom. Diaper creams act as a barrier between baby's skin and a potential irritant. Coconut oil is a natural antimicrobial and antifungal. It offers a nice layer of protection and sooths the skin. Trying different brands of laundry detergent (or disposable diapers) may also help with rashes.

29

Postpartum Depression — Moms and Dads

Moms and dads experience significant changes in their lives after childbirth, as they adjust to an array of new demands. Postnatal experiences can pose many challenges to both parents. Life feels much easier when you're happy. Finding ways to openly discuss mental health and well-being, especially postpartum blues or depression, will help you to find ways to address any underlying feelings.

Baby Blues

Signs and symptoms of baby blues can vary, lasting from a few days to a couple of weeks. Baby blues are milder, less severe than depression, and fade on their own. They often include some of the following signs:

- Mood swings
- Anxiety
- Sadness
- Irritability
- Feeling overwhelmed
- Crying

- Reduced concentration
- Appetite problems
- Trouble sleeping

It is normal to experience these feelings for a short while after childbirth. Around 80% of new mothers report this short-term decline in mood. Many mothers feel overwhelmed and irritable from a lack of sleep, and decreasing hormone levels. Having a baby is a big change in your life, and you are likely to feel much better by the time your baby is a week or two old. If your feelings and overall decline in mood lasts for a much longer period, you may be experiencing postpartum depression.

Postpartum Depression Symptoms

Postpartum depression is more intense and lasts longer than baby blues. Experiencing symptoms of depression may interfere with your ability to care for your newborn, or cope with other daily tasks. It is important to understand that feeling depressed is not a character flaw. Postpartum depression signs and symptoms may include:

- Severe mood swings
- Struggling to bonding with your baby
- Withdrawal from friends, support systems or family
- Trouble sleeping or sleeping too much
- Overwhelming fatigue
- A lack of enjoyment and interest in activities that you used to take pleasure in
- Intense irritability and anger
- Fear that you're not a good mother
- Hopelessness
- Feelings of worthlessness, shame, guilt or inadequacy
- Severe anxiety and panic attacks

- Thoughts of harming yourself or your baby

For moms, untreated postpartum depression can last for months and become a disorder. For dads, postpartum depression can cause an emotional strain for everyone close to a new baby. When a new mother is depressed, the risk of depression in the baby's father may increase.

Risk Factors and Causes

Physical and emotional changes may cause postpartum depression. Following childbirth, a mother experiences a significant drop in estrogen and progesterone. This can leave you feeling tired, down and lacking energy. You may feel less attractive, or struggling for a sense of individual identity, while being overwhelmed with newborn care. If you are not feeling like yourself, I encourage you to reach out to your partner, support systems or medical caregiver.

Risk Factors

1. Stress at home or at work
2. Financial issues
3. Frequent feelings of being overwhelmed
4. History of family depression
5. Postpartum depression after a previous pregnancy
6. Complications during pregnancy, traumatic or premature birth
7. Relationship problems with your partner or family

Treatment, Coping, and Support

Postpartum depression can be managed and treated. Professional help and making some changes to your daily life can help you recover quicker. Talk to your doctor, support groups and other new moms or women that have postpartum depression. Gathering support makes it easier to work through any feelings, allowing you to get back to enjoying time with your baby.

Lifestyle changes

1. **Healthy lifestyle** —adopt a nutrient rich diet. **Omega-3 acids** (found in Cod liver oil, salmon, walnuts, and avocado) and **Vitamin B** are proven energy and mood boosters. **Exercise** as part of your daily routine. Outdoor walks with your baby are a great way to stay physically active and de-stress. **Keep hydrated.**
2. **Babywearing**—a practice of transporting your baby in a carrier to promote bonding.
3. **Set practical expectations** — adjust your expectations of the "perfect" household. Complete your daily routine only as you can, and leave the rest for when you can manage. **Ask for help** and let people know when you require help.
4. **Make time for yourself** — adequately **rest and sleep** as much as you can. Spend time outside of the house, engaged with hobbies, or have some alone time with your partner or friends.
5. Things can get serious; don't forget to **laugh!**
6. **Acupuncture**— it is deeply healing, while also reduces anxiety and stress.
7. If you are experiencing postpartum depression, make an appointment to **see your doctor** or healthcare provider.

Taking care of your newborn also includes taking care of yourself.

30

Self-Love and Self-Awareness

You have entered a new and exciting phase of your life as a parent! The future is bright with many adventures, and new opportunities, for both you and your child. Almost every parent has a deep desire to entice their children into a life that is much more delicious, rewarding, and sweeter than their own. We strive to empower our children with tools to live successful, happy, healthy, and remarkable lives.

Yet even our utmost intentions can unintentionally hurt, disturb, and misalign our children from experiencing *their* best version of life. This phase may be daunting, but that should not deter you from finding ways to put your best self forward, for your children. You are ready to put into practice your natural and learned parental abilities!

Looking Good and Feeling Bad

Many children live in circumstances where they gradually give up, or lose, a little piece of their unique personality each day. Parents may inflict their own hopes and dreams on their children. We desperately try to make our children perform in a perfect role. This role is often solely created by us, and shaped by the need to fulfill desires we haven't achieved ourselves.

Losing your self-image does not occur overnight. It is a gradual process that can follow us well into adulthood. At first, it goes unnoticed in the early stages of childhood. As children we unquestioningly accept opinions, submit to schedules, and try to meet expectations. We exchange others' ideas in place of our own, and learn to become people-pleasers, especially for our parents. Children are aware that their survival depends on the adults that care for them. In order to fit within an ambitious plan, children participate in activities and do whatever is necessary to find a place in the world around them.

At this early point, there is a division within the child—on one hand, to follow a deeper yearning from an inner voice, or on the other, to please a parent. By ignoring this inner voice, we learn to abandon our true nature. While it is a process for children to feel like they fit in, feel safe, and feel accepted, not all conscious choices feel right within the child. Moving towards someone else's path moves you away from own path.

Once the connection to your true self is lost, you are left with an artificial connection to the world. We become extrinsically (externally) driven, and are often left searching for answers later in life. As parents, our hope should be to create an environment that will foster the unique character and abilities of each of our children. We should aspire to support our children with their choices, all in their own time and in their own way. This type of environment will reinforce the self-esteem of a child, and help them pursue their interpretation of a best life.

The strength of our self-esteem largely determines the quality of our life. Intrinsic (internal) motivation is a powerful tool for self-fulfillment. Being internally rewarded continually reminds us of how amazing and capable we are. Strong self-esteem helps define a clear boundary between people pleasing or self-betrayal, and true empathy or love. It reminds us that all the qualities we seek are, in fact, and always have been, present within us.

Truth is a bridge between the mind and the heart. It allows us to genuinely and honestly explore who we are, and to express ourselves. As you have discovered in this process of growth, staying true to your desires is the path to successful outcomes.

Change Is Constant

We grow from all experiences, especially circumstances that push our core disposition. Many changes occur out of our control, and even against our will. The nature of change is constant, and age is only a measure of how far we have moved forward through our inescapable human experience. We are unlike most other creatures on our planet, who can take their first steps almost immediately after birth. As humans, we experience many levels of growth over time. Even as adults, when we are physically strong enough to leave the nest, we continue to be stuck in roles and experiences that contribute towards our growth.

Our world is beautiful, full of wonder and awe. But it is multi-dimensional, and our full experience will always include recessions, catastrophic events, or unhappy people. A stable and happy home creates an environment for a child to grow while feeling confident, understood, and secure. A healthy environment allows children to creatively and safely expresses their deepest thoughts and feelings. This foundation is empowering, and it gives our children the best opportunity to navigate through the human experience.

Our journey has shown us that all growth is by choice. We can become the composer of our own life story at any time we choose. Everything we need is within ourselves. Once we discover that faith, love, hope, peace, and happiness are always present in our hearts, we will never be limited in the same way again.

Love is a force that nurtures and upholds our children with respect. Love allows us to embrace our children's fresh views and ideas, fostering their comfort and protection. Your depth of love has been wildly unleashed, and you are daringly deeply in love with your newborn. In this awakening, you have discovered an inner home, where you feel a sense of purpose and belonging. You feel peace, when you are at peace with who you are. You feel joy, when you truly enjoy who you are. You feel unconditional love, when you are a parent. I wish you a happy and fulfilling life.

"Your children are not your children.
They are the sons and daughters of Life's longing for itself.
They come through you but not from you,
And though they are with you, yet they belong not to you.
You may give them your love but not your thoughts,
For they have their own thoughts.
You may house their bodies but not their souls,
For their souls dwell in the house of tomorrow,
Which you cannot visit, not even in your dreams."

—Kahlil Gibran

Lucy Bare is a Wellness Coach and Birth Doula. She offers practical and inspired coaching using a combination of healing techniques to achieve clarity, and restore confidence in all areas of your life.

Lucy's website is here: https://www.lucybare.com/

Under pen name "Lucy Bear" she has released:

- A pocket guide to your pregnancy: Become Your Own Doula
- A Winding Road to the Heart
- Life Does Not Need Your Consent
- Between the Earth and Stars
- In Pursuit of your Magic: A Wellness Workbook

We are unlike most other creatures on our planet, who can take their first steps almost immediately after birth. As humans, we experience many levels of growth over time. Even as adults, when we are physically strong enough to leave the nest, we continue to encounter situations and relationships that challenge us beyond our limits. Lucy's work as a Wellness Coach and Birth Doula is dedicated to respect and value Humans as precious Beings.

www.ingramcontent.com/pod-product-compliance
Lightning Source LLC
Chambersburg PA
CBHW051438290426
44109CB00016B/1604